MIGRAINE

What Works!

MIGRAINE
What Works!

A Complete Guide to Overcoming
and Preventing Migraines

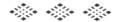

Revised 2nd Edition

JOSEPH KANDEL, **M.D.**
DAVID B. SUDDERTH, **M.D.**

PRIMA PUBLISHING

Special thanks go to Chris Adamec for her extensive assistance. Also thanks to Betty Lavery for her dedicated persistence in transcription. We especially acknowledge Sue Felber for her insightful assistance in obtaining relevant resources for our research, and our devoted office staff for their patience during the writing and production of this book.

Published by Prima Publishing, Roseville, California. Member of the Crown Publishing Group, a division of Random House, Inc.

PRIMA PUBLISHING and colophon are trademarks of Random House, Inc., registered with the United States Patent and Trademark Office.

WARNING—DISCLAIMER
This book is not intended to replace medical guidance. Persons under doctors' care for headaches should consult with their physicians. Responsibility for any adverse effects resulting from the use of information in this book rests solely with the reader.

Library of Congress Cataloging-in-Publication
Kandel, Joseph.
    Migraine—what works! : a complete guide to overcoming and preventing migraines / Joseph Kandel and David B. Sudderth.—2nd. ed.
        p. cm.
    Includes bibliographical references and index.
    ISBN 0-7615-2143-7
    1. Migraine—Popular works.   I. Sudderth, David B.   II. Title.
RC392.K36   2000
616.8'57—dc21   99-049742
                                                                CIP
01 02 03 04 HH 10 9 8 7 6 5 4 3 2
Printed in the United States of America

Second Edition

Visit us online at www.primapublishing.com

To my wife, Merrylee, and our children, Max, Hannah Rose, and Geena. Your love, patience, and support made this work possible. And to my parents, for their unending love.

JOSEPH KANDEL

To my friends, family, patients, and teachers, without whose interest and encouragement this work would not have been possible.

DAVID B. SUDDERTH

CONTENTS

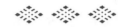

INTRODUCTION

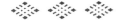

Migraine is a common, cruel, and pervasive disorder suffered by 23 million Americans, not only afflicting them with great pain but also robbing them of control over their personal, family, and work lives. The National Center for Health Statistics reports that migraine headaches result in a loss of 30 million work days costing the economy $4.5 billion per year. Further, no one could begin to accurately quantify the collective anguish and pain migraineurs suffer, as well as their loss of personal and professional opportunities. Yet today there is much hope for migraineurs, thanks to new treatment and medication.

People have suffered from migraines since recorded time. The ancient Babylonians, Greeks, and Romans experienced migraines, and cave dwellers probably did, too. Famous individuals, including Thomas Jefferson, Alexander Pope, Dorothy Wordsworth, Ulysses S. Grant, and many others were migraine sufferers. According to Grant's own memoirs, one of his migraines evaporated upon the news of Lee's surrender.

The pain of these famous migraine sufferers of the past was no more intense than the suffering of today's enterprising computer programmer, civil servant, or any other individual with an agonizing migraine. But there is one difference: today physicians can alleviate much of that pain. It's rare for a neurologist to be completely unable to assist the patient with debilitating migraine headaches. As physicians, we are very optimistic about the prognosis for migraineurs, and you should be, too!

1

What Is a Migraine?

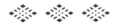

A migraine is a serious, debilitating, and often painful illness originating in the brain. The migraine may last for a few minutes or a few days—or for any period of time in between.

Subtypes of Migraine

Migraine headaches are divided into two major subtypes: the classic migraine and the common migraine. The key difference between the two is that the classic migraine follows an "aura," while a common migraine appears with no aura.

So what's an aura? The aura is a brief episode of symptoms that are related to a focal area of dysfunction in the brain and may include visual disturbances, dizziness, and other symptoms. The aura will be discussed in greater detail later in this chapter.

Sometimes people with classic migraine also suffer from common migraine. Getting one kind doesn't exempt you from getting the other form. Sorry!

In order to diagnose and treat migraines, we adhere to the headache classification committee guidelines of the International Headache Society.

FREQUENCY OF OCCURRENCE

People who experience common migraine headaches usually suffer from one to four headaches per month. Yet about 10% have ten or more migraines monthly, and some people have no more than two to three attacks of migraine in their entire lives.

Common migraine is seen more often by doctors, occurs more frequently, and lasts longer than does the classic migraine. Nausea and vomiting are also worse in the common migraine. All this doesn't necessarily mean that classic migraine is "better"—it's not the one you'd choose if you could pick one over the other. Classic migraine has its own scary elements, notably the aura aspect, which we'll discuss in a few pages.

MIGRAINE DIFFERS FROM PERSON TO PERSON

One fact that may surprise you is that the onset and the course of the illness varies greatly among "migraineurs" (people who suffer from migraines), and some people—not very many!—don't even get a headache. This chapter discusses what actually happens to the body during an acute attack. Let's start off with an interesting but unusual case.

Anne B., 35, came to the office with very peculiar symptoms, primarily involving recurring "black eyes." She was mystified. The black eyes were spontaneous—they "just happened" and didn't seem to be associated with any other symptoms.

Intermittent headaches had been a serious problem for Anne for several years, but in the past twelve months, her headaches had changed and, unfortunately, had become considerably worse. These new headaches would begin as an aching type of headache and within thirty minutes would surge into excruciating pain, intense nausea, and vomiting.

Often the "raccoon eyes" were present the day after one of these severe headaches, although Anne said that the eye discoloration could occur before the headaches or even with no headache.

The black eye symptoms Anne experienced are only one of the many physical changes that may occur in a patient with migraine. We treated Anne with a moderate dose of Inderal along with intermittent Sumatriptan, and she has greatly improved with regard to her headache frequency and duration.

Profound alterations may also occur in the circulatory system, gastrointestinal function, and mental and emotional states of the patient. In fact, some of the phenomena witnessed in a migrainous attack belong to the most fascinating and exciting realm of human existence.

If you suffer from migraine, you probably know that this illness is enthralling to some medical observers and irksome and perplexing to others. You also know that the various features of the migraine attack can often lead to intense and excruciating misery in the patient. Some patients are driven into a desperate panic or a bewildered lethargic state.

The bottom line: It's no fun at all.

Prodrome

Sometimes migraineurs get a kind of advance warning of an impending migraine, a sort of "yellow light" alert, which is called the "prodrome."

A prodrome is different from an aura because the prodromal symptoms may be very vague and begin slowly, with great variation in how long they last. Vague warnings of an impending headache often precede either the headache or the aura, and if sufferers can take immediate action, they may be able to stop the migraine cold—or at least beat it back to a bearable level.

Prodromes occur more frequently than the aura itself does. Comments such as "I don't feel myself today" and "I feel like a train hit me"—along with many other remarks ranging between both extremes—are common from migraineurs prior to the onslaught of their headaches. It should also be emphasized here that occasionally a prodrome will not develop into a full-blown migrainous attack.

Changes in mood are common prodromal symptoms; for example, patients may feel very depressed and lethargic. But sometimes, they actually feel a sense of increased well-being and a high energy level. But watch out! Bad times lie ahead as the migraine comes on like a speeding bullet.

Felix S., 32, our patient for several years, was diagnosed as having common migrainous attacks, which were fairly well controlled with Inderal. The additional use of injectable Sumatriptan has greatly helped reduce the severity of his attacks.

Felix says that he always knew when a headache was coming the second he opened his eyes in the morning. He could barely lift himself out of bed, and once he was finally out, he was intensely irritable. His family knew to stay out of his way.

THE AURA

Migraine sufferers may also experience a range of symptoms classified under an experience known as the "aura."

The aura is a brief episode of symptoms that are related to a focal area of dysfunction in the brain. In general, an aura lasts less than twenty minutes and usually appears before the head pain begins. However, the aura can recur at various points of the headache, such as during the most intensely painful point.

Auras may be simple (migraineurs see flashing lights, wavy lines, etc.) or have the character of a complex hallucinatory experience—truly frightening. However, once the nature of the aura has been carefully explained to and understood by the migraineur, its more horrifying aspects can be dispelled.

Visual Aura

Visual auras are the most common among those who experience any form of aura. The more simple visual disturbance is the "photopsia," which consists of circles, triangles, squares, or other geometric patterns, usually white or multicolored. Typically, the person sees these figures in any part of the visual field, and they may move about. Although not really there, the patterns are clearly "seen" by the migraineur. This may be due to irritation to the vision center of the brain and probably has nothing to do with either eye.

Sometimes more complex and symmetrical patterns are occasionally seen. These visual disturbances may occur even if the person is blind or both eyes have been physically removed. Here is one description given by a migraine sufferer, quoted by Sacks in the medical book, *Migraine— Evolution of a Common Disorder* (University of California Press, 1970):

> a bright stellate object, a small angled sphere suddenly appears in one side of the combined field . . . it rapidly enlarges . . . and, as the increase in size goes on, the outline here becomes broken, the gap becoming larger as the hole increases, and the original circular outline

becomes oval . . . when this angled oval has extended through the greater part of the half-field the upper portion expands; it seems to overcome at least some resistance in the immediate neighborhood of the fixing point . . . so that a bulge occurs in the part above, and the angular elements of the outline here enlarge. . . . This final expansion near the centre progresses with great rapidity, and ends a whirling centre of light from which sprays of light seem flying off. Then all is over, and the headache comes on.

That sounds bad enough, but some patients have also reported truly complex and bizarre visual disturbances—so unsettling they were reluctant to report them to their doctors unless specifically asked about them. Why? Probably because they feared their doctors would consider them mentally ill. But neurologists are very familiar with this problem and need to be told what's going on so they can help you.

Another example of visual aura is when an object is seen as extremely distorted, much like images and proportions are distorted in a funhouse mirror. An Alice in Wonderland experience can occur where suddenly a person may appear to have an elongated neck or someone's head may appear dramatically larger while the legs looks disproportionately small.

Changes in distance perceptions may occur, too—how close or how far away objects appear to be may be completely out of alignment with reality. Think of the warning on the sideview mirror on some cars: "Objects in mirror are closer than they appear." Then magnify that ten times or more.

Disorders of sensation and movement are the next most common features of a classic aura. Often the sensation may involve a feeling of numbness on one side of the face, usually the mouth, and also in the hand and arm on the same side of the body. These symptoms tend to develop within thirty minutes and can terrify the patient, who is convinced that he or she is in the middle of a stroke or maybe even dying.

Weakness or clumsiness in the arms and legs often occur as part of the aura. Sometimes pain in a limb is the primary feature of an aura.

Other Types of Aura

Dizziness or abnormal sensations of motion are well-documented features of an aura. Other hallucinatory experiences can consist of auditory misperceptions, such as a ringing or crackling noise in the ears.

Sometimes patients will lose the ability to speak (aphasia), although comprehension of spoken language usually is not lost. Or they may experience an olfactory hallucination, where they smell something that is not there. Fortunately, both aphasia and olfactory hallucinations are rarely reported. Often migraineurs have a sensation of "deja vu," that they are re-experiencing feelings or sensations exactly as they have in the past.

In one reported case, a 38-year-old man who suffered from severe migraines also usually experienced amnesia during the attacks. However, at one point he reported that he did remember seeing gray Indians, 20 centimeters high, crowding around him in his room. This most likely represented an irritation in the part of the brain that handles memory. Such an irritation affects certain fibers that pass through this area carrying or triggering vision sensations.

THE HEADACHE

The headache can be absent altogether, or it can be so agonizingly painful that the patient seriously contemplates suicide. Often the headache is on one side (called hemicranial—

half of the head), but it can occur on both sides of the head. Sometimes the sides even switch! The left side could suddenly become pain-free and then the right side is in agony (or vice versa). Headaches that occur on only one side seem to be more painful.

The initial pain of a migraine is often described as vise-like or of a pressing, gripping nature that may later progress to a throbbing, banging, or pounding headache.

The migrainous head pain can be localized to anywhere on the face or scalp and can even affect the structures of the upper portion of the neck. Usually, the frontal (forehead) regions are affected, as well as the eye area.

Pain may affect the person's entire skull, and the scalp itself is often very tender during a migrainous attack. Sometimes the migraine is confined to the lower area of the face below the eyes and is called a lower-half migraine.

Most migraines last from one to three hours, although children sometimes experience headaches of less than ten minutes.

The migraine is so devastating to the body that few sufferers can think of anything but the pain and suffering. In addition, activities which increase the pressure inside the brain—such as sneezing, coughing, or vomiting—can be agonizingly painful to the patient. Often migraineurs press on the pulsating arteries in front of their ears, trying to control the pain. This usually doesn't work.

OTHER SYMPTOMS

If cigarette smoke or perfume bothers you when you have a migraine, you are not alone. Often virtually any odor is intolerable to migraineurs, and strong odors can increase the physical pain of the headache.

Sometimes loud noises disturb the person with a migraine; this is often referred to as phonophobia. No drumrolls, please, and make your teenager use headphones.

Likewise, bright lights or even routine daylight can increase your pain. This is called photophobia.

Nausea and Vomiting

About half of all patients suffer from nausea and vomiting. Sometimes the arrival of nausea signals that the head pain will abate; however, it could also mean the pain is going to get worse! The significance of nausea and vomiting truly varies from person to person, and people who suffer from migraines learn what it means from their own experience. Generally, nausea signals that things are going to get better or they're going to get worse, rather than stay the same.

Sometimes the vomiting is so severe or the person sweats so much that he or she loses too much fluid and needs intravenous therapy to replace the loss of water and sodium. Conversely, sometimes fluid is retained in the body.

Gastrointestinal changes include diarrhea or constipation and abdominal cramps. In addition to these abdominal changes, one of the most significant aspects migraine sufferers experience is that, at the time of an acute attack, the stomach can actually become paralyzed. That's right, they can encounter what's called "gastroparesis," which complicates the migraine even more by preventing medicines taken by mouth from being effective. Since oral medications have to go through the stomach to work, it makes sense that other forms of intervention may be necessary. This is an all-too-often overlooked aspect of migraine management, particularly by physicians who are not comfortable providing care to migraineurs.

Intervention in the form of medications by nasal spray, rectal suppository, or injection may become the medication of choice to abort an acute migraine, particularly if the migraine has been present for more than thirty to sixty minutes. This is the approximate time frame it takes for the stomach to become sluggish or even stop absorbing chemicals, nutrients, and medications.

Circulatory Changes

In the beginning of this chapter, we described the patient with the "raccoon eyes," which apparently resulted from circulatory changes associated with her migraines.

More frequently, we see patients who are very pale, except for flushing that may be seen on one side of the face— the hurting side. Sometimes the dilation of blood vessels is so severe that it causes actual hemorrhage (severe bleeding) in the nose area, or superficially in the eyeballs.

Increased blood flow in the mucous membranes of the nose can also cause nasal congestion, drooping eyelids, and changes in eye pupil sizes. It can lead to sinus congestion and is often related to that stuffy sensation of the nose, which can be confused with sinusitis.

The patient may insist that he or she has a fever when there is no fever, while others complain they feel cold and clammy, especially in their hands and feet.

The heart rate may increase or decrease in this multifaceted illness.

Changes in Behavior

If the greatest and most heartfelt wish of the migraineur is relief from headache, the second greatest wish is for seclusion. Just leave them alone!

Unlike patients with kidney stones or cluster headaches, who characteristically rush about or leave home seeking relief, the migraineur will generally choose an immobile position. Usually migraine victims will lie down, although they may sit or stand very still.

Patients in the throes of an uncomfortable attack are generally very irritable, although some may be passive. People who are normally even-tempered, kind, and loving individuals can be transformed into stubborn, rude, and extremely insensitive creatures.

One patient told us that during an attack, he looked like a wax statue, felt like a martyr, and behaved like Satan himself.

Sometimes people with migraine become extremely drowsy and all they want to do is sleep. It's not a good idea to try to wake them up! Let sleeping migraineurs lie.

Mental ability can even be affected by a migraine. Patients with migraines generally perform more poorly than they normally would on tests requiring higher-ordered processes such as mathematical thought, concentration, or creative activity. In addition, memory lapses may occur, and the unhappy and perplexed migraineur may later be confronted with things he or she said or did during an attack—but doesn't remember at all.

Sometimes behavioral changes are extreme, and in very rare cases can even be psychotic. For example, the patient may feel a sense of unreality or may become violent and uncontrollable and need to be restrained, either chemically or physically. Patients who react in this way during migraine episodes usually don't remember what happened during the attack.

It's Over . . . For Now

As the migraine subsides and ends, most patients state that they still don't feel "right." Often, they complain of a lack of initiative, a kind of mental dullness or cloudiness and a generalized weakness. One patient said she feels "like a zombie" after an attack. After such a massive assault on the body that some migraine headaches cause, this reaction is certainly not surprising.

So far we have attempted to describe the symptoms of migraine from the simple to the complex. What type of process can lead to such a bizarre and variable collection of symptoms? In the next chapter, we will explore the leading theories offered to account for this truly perplexing disorder.

....

2

....

THEORIES OF MIGRAINE: WHAT CAUSES THEM?

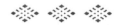

What actually causes people to suffer from migraine headaches? Physicians aren't entirely sure, but they do have theories for the basic causes. Most doctors generally select from four primary theories.

You don't need to become a medical doctor to understand these theories, and it's a good idea to learn what physicians believe is the likely cause of your problem. Why? Because knowledge is power, and the more you understand your own body and your reactions to food and medications, the more you are empowered to combat the insidious problem of migraine headaches.

One type of migraine, basilar migraine, can actually appear as a coma. Therefore, it is important for your doctor to understand the variety of migraine disorders and how they manifest themselves. This knowledge will often provide clues to help determine what underlies the migraine.

We can classify theories of migraine causes as:

- Vascular
- Neural

- Neurovascular (a combination of neural and vascular)
- Neurochemical transmission/depletion theory

THE VASCULAR THEORY OF MIGRAINE

Clinicians who support the vascular theory believe that a migraine headache results directly from the expansion and contraction of blood vessels, both inside *and* outside the brain. When blood vessels dilate outside the brain, says this theory, this causes the blood vessels inside the brain to constrict.

Along with the narrowing of the blood vessels inside the brain comes a decreased blood flow and diminished oxygen flow to structures inside your brain. As a result of these changes, neurological symptoms such as migraines occur. Or so the theory goes.

Over the past decade, research has documented actual changes in blood flow during both the prodrome and onset of a migraine episode. Initially, with the spasm of blood vessels, there is also a change in the blood flow to the brain, and the migraine aura theoretically results from this spasm.

Then the blood dilations expand, and a release of numerous chemicals, known as vasoactive substances, occurs. This release is often associated with the "pounding" sensation from which migraine patients suffer.

The sequence continues, as the release of those vasoactive substances apparently triggers some central mechanism that lowers the pain threshold. That means it hurts you more than it would otherwise because your pain tolerance is decreased.

Additional evidence and anecdotal references do support the "pulsing temples," referring to the blood vessels over the forehead. These do actually appear to pulsate in a number of patients during a migraine episode.

In further support, in some cases, migraines can be treated by firm pressure over the temples, and some physicians have suggested constricting headband-like devices as curative.

More recently, using a device called a transcranial doppler (which monitors blood flow through the brain and arteries), researchers have found that the speed of blood flow in the middle cerebral artery decreases during a migraine attack. Somehow, your brain turns on the "yellow light" and the blood flow slows down, which is bad for migraineurs.

Further support for this theory comes from the fact that, in many cases, medications used to treat or prevent migraines specifically act by affecting the blood vessel wall stability. Such medications include beta blockers: Inderal, Tenormin, and Corgard. In addition, first-line medications for treating migraines have included calcium channel blockers such as Calan SR, Procardia, and Cardizem, which may act in a similar way.

Research done in 1995, using very specialized techniques of blood flow measurement, has revealed that during classic migraine, there is a region of a progressive decrease in blood flow. This is a key to the blood flow theory of migraine, and draws a relationship to migraines and "ischemic" strokes (related to lack of blood and oxygen).

Other researchers have concluded that there may be some association between the blood flow events of migraine and a future connection with the loss of blood and oxygen to the brain, resulting in stroke. The results were not clear-cut, but certainly do lend credence to the vascular theory of migraine disorder.

THE NEURAL THEORY

The neural hypothesis takes a slightly different approach to the causes of migraine headache disorders. Supporters of this theory believe that a migraine is actually a dysfunction of the nervous system and an unstable threshold in the brain.

When internal or external stressors increase, this threshold is exceeded, and a migraine headache is produced. It's sort of like one part of your body says "don't step over this line," but you do anyway, and suffer the consequences (all unconsciously, of course!).

This theory also seems to rely on a belief that there is a genetic predisposition for migraine headache disorders. It is true that migraine sufferers often have a strong family history of migraine. To further the theory of a genetic predisposition toward migraine, one sophisticated study found that a location on chromosome 19 was related to a unique type of migraine.

Another aspect of the neural theory is the belief that migraine is comprised of a unique constellation of symptoms, one of which is often misdiagnosed since it is too tough for the average primary care doc to call.

It's believed, as part of this theory, that migraine results from an irregular or abnormal nervous system outflow, a burst of electric energy, which can kindle or trigger a variety of areas in the brain. This subsequently produces a variety of symptoms, sort of like a microscopic lightning strike inside your brain.

As a result, many diverse symptoms may occur, such as severe headache associated with nausea and vomiting. Hallucinations may also occur, including imagined sights, sounds, tastes, or even smells. In addition, the patient may experience a variation of migraine that is also associated with abdominal queasiness often referred to as "abdominal migraine."

This theory also explains changes in mood or behavior, such as an essentially untriggered sense of elation, depression, anger, increased or decreased libido, or hunger—all of which can be symptoms of irritation in various parts of the brain.

In addition, imbalance and unsteadiness and even weakness and numbness can often be ascribed to atypical migraines.

Documented studies have also revealed that during the migraine phase, there are imbalances of glucose mechanism in different parts of the brain, suggesting that various parts of the brain are "selectively vulnerable" for certain people. This may explain why there is a tendency for one side of the head versus the other to become involved during migraine attacks.

In "complicated migraine," patients may present with weakness, numbness, language or speech dysfunction, and clumsiness and unsteadiness, depending on which parts of the brain are affected at a given time. These episodes can often mimic stroke symptoms and confuse physicians who are not neurologists. Yet, when the episode has subsided, within minutes to hours the neurological symptoms disappear as well.

As an example, psychiatrists have used the concept of "kindling" to explain causes of major depression. Frequently, the theory goes, there is irritation of a specific part of the brain (usually the temporal lobes) that can explain behavioral changes.

Similarly, once one part of the brain is kindled or the threshold is dropped, then other parts of the brain can likewise become irritable, and thus trigger chemical changes of the brain.

THE NEUROVASCULAR THEORY

Supporters of this theory take a combination approach, believing that during attacks migraineurs have both abnormal or unstable blood vessels combined with a nervous system irritability.

It appears that much of the skull or facial pain that patients experience during migraine is carried along the distribution of the trigeminovascular pathways. (The trigeminal nerve is located near the cheekbone.) A possible defect in the chemical discharge along this pathway appears to be what causes the problem.

Think of this pathway as the highway where messages of pain are sent through the brain stem and into the sensory receptor (thalamus) part of the brain.

The result of stimulation can be that additional messages are sent to areas of the brain that interpret pain. So various parts of your brain are all saying "I feel pain!" And you do.

Combined with this is the problem that the intracranial blood vessels become unstable, with subsequent spasm and expansion of the blood vessels. The spasm, which is actually a protective mechanism to alter blood flow within your brain, can produce the changes associated with a lack of blood and oxygen. This is often referred to as the "migraine aura" and thus is how the supporters of this theory explain the aura.

Taking this theory a little further, the messages, which are carried up through the brain stem fibers to the thalamus and on to the cerebral cortex (the thinking part of the brain), are then associated with a spreading wave of chemical changes throughout your thinking center. This is often referred to as the "spreading depression" of migraine. Depending on the size of the region involved, various neurological signs and symptoms may occur.

This theory does seem to explain why a small number of patients have a multitude of symptoms without the clear-cut headache of migraine. In fact, the area of the brain that is involved with this spreading depression apparently determines which symptoms a patient may experience.

For example, if the motor cortex were affected, then a patient might be weak or clumsy in an arm or leg or one side of the body only. On the other hand, if the frontal lobe regions became involved, a patient may feel confused, disoriented. and experience impaired judgment, feeling like he or she is "in a fog."

This unified hypothesis has been supported by various clinical studies, which have also revealed that a number of chemicals play a role in the brain stem function, including serotonin and acetylcholine—although serotonin is probably the major player.

In a domino-like effect, activation of nerve cells in a region of the brain stem (the locus ceruleus), as well as in the dorsal raphe nuclei of the brain stem, apparently triggers a response in the nerve cells and the supporting structures and blood vessels of the region. All these responses taken together trigger an inflammatory response within the brain tissue itself, often through the trigeminal vascular pathways.

Throughout this whole process of body reactions and changes, there also appears to be a rebound effect, which seems to continue with the pain/inflammatory response. Compare it to a floodgate opening up. Not just one drop of water drips out, but instead all the water in the dam pours out.

Similarly, once the neurovascular system is inflamed, the neurochemicals or vasoactive substances that are released can continue a cycle of allowing the brain stem and thalamus to acknowledge pain and irritability, thereby keeping up the pain syndrome long after the external cause has been removed.

Since trigger causes are an important part of this theory, physicians who support it believe that patients should try to avoid those substances that apparently trigger migraine within their bodies. Some commonly known triggers are certain foods, such as cheese, citrus fruits, or chocolate, and some chemical food additives such as MSG.

In addition, stress, heat, infections, fumes, hormonal changes, and menstrual cycles can trigger migraines.

Note: Of course, hormonal changes and menstrual cycles are not so easily avoided. Some physicians have suggested women who suffer from migraine headaches during menstruation can mitigate the problem by taking an NSAID medication for five days before the cycle and also during the cycle. Others recommend that the patient take amitriptyline or propranolol during their menses. There is also some evidence that percutaneous estradiol gel just before and during menstruation can reduce the incidence of migraines.

Other triggers can be lack of sleep, too much sleep, or missing a meal. Drugs, including alcohol, can be powerful triggers for migraines. Weather changes can also trigger a migraine headache.

Neurochemical Transmission/Depletion: The Serotonin Theory

A growing volume of research literature supports the role of impaired communication (neurotransmission) between brain cells (neurons). The brain is a telecommunications system *par excellence,* relying not only on electrical events but chemical occurrences as well to modulate the behavior of other cells. Serotonin is one of the many chemical neurotransmitters involved in intercellular communication (communication between brain cells). The serotonin-mediated chemical pathways are clearly implicated in the perception of pain.

Possibly the most supportive evidence is patient response to medications affecting serotonin. Many patients experience great relief from migraines by taking medications that directly affect serotonin levels, most notably Imitrex.

Researchers have recorded decreased blood levels of serotonin during migraine episodes, and urine concentrations of serotonin breakdown products seems to increase, so it is clear that there are serotonin changes in the body during a migraine headache. Some medications can also cause migraines. It appears as though medications that may reduce the circulating volume of serotonin may indeed trigger migraine episodes.

Additional support for this theory is that there are serotonin receptors in the stomach lining, which may explain why nausea and vomiting sometimes occur during an acute migraine attack.

Research in the 1970s and 1980s also revealed that implanting electrodes in the brain stem could produce migraine-like symptoms that lasted for days, weeks, months, or years. (Those poor research rats!) This coincides with the high concentration of serotonin receptors, which are presumed to control and modulate pain.

There are actually four different kinds of serotonin receptors. (Don't worry—we won't get too technical here!) Class one serotonin receptors appear to affect smooth muscle relaxation and smooth muscle contraction.

Class two serotonin receptors affect the discharge of nerve cells, the tightening of blood vessels, as well as some of the contraction to the airways in the lungs and the stomach wall.

Class three lead to activation of autonomic reflexes as well as to some nerve cell excitation in the brain and spinal cord.

Class four affect the stomach wall, heart stimulation, and relaxation of the food tube.

The serotonin theory explains why certain medications act on serotonin receptor one to block migraine episodes and relieve symptoms, while other medications work better on serotonin receptor two and so on.

Some people, especially holistic practitioners, are quick to point out that trace mineral changes in the body, vitamin deficiencies, and borderline nutrient deficiencies can all lead to severe migraine disorders. These practitioners approach headache disorders from that standpoint.

We feel that a combined theory of neurochemical changes (with an underlying genetic predisposition) lead to the cascade effect and the dumping of chemical changes in the brain, which lead to a vascular process—these best explain migraine now. This means that chemicals such as serotonin, norepinephrine, acetylcholine, GABA, and glutamate, among the many chemical messengers of the brain, reach some level of imbalance.

When the floodgates open, these chemicals irritate the blood vessels, and thus blood flow is altered. This change leads to the spreading change in oxygen and nutrients to various parts of the brain and explains the multitude of problems that migraine sufferers may experience. Depending upon which area of the brain is most vulnerable, we can see a variety of symptoms.

It is important to point out that when more than one theory exists regarding any medical problem, it means that no absolute answers are yet known. For example, in 1995, a new theory of migraine regarding a new tissue was proposed and reported in a popular magazine.

This tissue, heretofore unnoticed by physicians, was found at the base of the skull. The tissue was found by two dentists who were looking at causes of jaw pain and ended up cutting the skull of a cadaver at peculiar angles. Because of the change in dissection technique, this new tissue was discovered! The presumption is that this tissue, which is directly adjacent to the brain covering, can become very inflamed and can then trigger many responses, which in turn lead to headache pains similar to migraine disorder.

This is exciting, because it reveals that we are constantly gaining new information about how our bodies work and hopefully will eventually be able to put this information into one cohesive theory to explain the cause of migraine headache disorders.

MECHANISM OF MIGRAINE HEADACHE DISORDER

The mechanism of migraine headache disorder formation is an additional important concept of how migraines are produced. The theory, backed up by scientific studies, is that the migraine can be caused by a deficiency of certain trace elements and minerals.

As we discuss elsewhere in this book, such things as deficiency in magnesium are often related to severe migraine pains. Thus treatment with either magnesium through the vein or magnesium replacement by mouth can lead to reduction or complete cessation of the migraine headache. While this does not give the absolute mechanism, one can infer that deficiencies affect the chemical change either in the brain or on the blood vessel wall and therefore act as a gatekeeper for toxins.

When the deficiencies of magnesium or other trace minerals and elements are not available to your body, the natural gatekeeper is not there and thus toxins and pollutants can trigger a migraine headache disorder. We are learning new information regarding magnesium and other minerals and elements every day, and this gives hope for the future of new and rational approaches to the management of migraine headache pain.

Recently, new information has come to light about headaches as one symptom of a larger disease. For example, patients who have had liver transplants may actually suffer from a new onset of migraines. While these patients had been susceptible to underlying medical processes, such as hypertension, infections, and other illnesses due to the medications they had taken, they also developed a migraine headache syndrome.

Research on this phenomenon may reveal to us that there is a systemic connection with the different organ systems, and that these organ systems are tied in together into a feedback system for the central nervous system (brain, spinal cord, etc.).

What this means is that when one organ system is unwell, it may trigger a negative response and produce illness in other organ systems. This then may be the mechanism which is at play in patients who have had liver transplants and suffer new onset migraine disorders.

Sometimes it's difficult for physicians to diagnose migraines. Or what they do diagnose as a migraine headache is in fact another form of head pain.

3

Chronic Daily Headache and Other Causes of Headache Pain: If It's Not Migraine, Then What Is It?

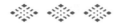

This chapter is one of the most important of this book. We will discuss the phenomenon of chronic daily headaches, which is a particularly distressing syndrome experienced by many migraine sufferers. We will also discuss some of the recent, disturbing reports about serious hazards of chronic use of over-the-counter medications.

Since there is some confusion between chronic daily headaches and migraine, a careful diagnosis is important. Remember, patients don't report in to the neurologist's office with the diagnosis "migraine" indelibly stamped on their foreheads. Instead, it takes the doctor some time, testing, and good professional judgment to make a determination.

The conditions discussed in this chapter are only the primary diagnostic entities that a qualified headache practitioner will consider in terms of a headache severe enough to warrant medical evaluation. Many are of a benign nature, but others can cause death.

Commonly recognized headache syndromes include muscle contraction headaches; temporomandibular joint dysfunction; neck disorders; trigeminal neuralgia; occipital neuralgia; eye disease; pseudotumor cerebri; cluster headaches; head trauma; temporal arteritis; tumors; abnormal blood vessels; stroke; and toxic states.

Chronic Daily Headaches

The chronic daily headache syndrome is a particularly distressing consequence of poorly treated migraine. While most neurologists are very familiar with this syndrome, many other physicians who treat migraine are grievously ignorant concerning the cause, nature, and treatment of this syndrome.

The syndrome consists of frequent headaches, usually for more than twenty days per month, in which the patient suffers from severe prostrating headaches, often accompanied by other common features of migraine. The pain can be entirely debilitating and lead to dehydration and utter despair in the patient.

The syndrome develops in an insidious manner. For example, migraineurs frequently have other types of headaches besides their migraines. They tend to use their anti-migrainous medications to deal with the other headaches that occur more often.

Initially, these headaches tend to respond to the medication. But then greater amounts of the drug are required over time to have the same effect. The medication in question can be ergotamine, acetaminophen, aspirin, or many of the other medications used for migraine, including those containing the barbiturate butalbital.

As the medication wears off, a very predictable headache appears: the chronic daily headache pattern. Interestingly, this type of headache pattern does not occur in non-migraineurs who actually take similar amounts and types of medication. For example, the syndrome is virtually unknown in patients suffering solely from cluster headaches or in arthritic patients who take large amounts of these medications.

It has also been shown from various studies that the antidepressant amitriptyline (Elavil), which is of great benefit as a preventive medication, is rendered ineffective in this context—more isn't better for the migraineur with daily headaches. Yet once the cycle of nearly daily headaches is broken, amitriptyline again becomes quite helpful in preventing not only migraines, but the other headaches from which migraineurs frequently suffer.

The severity and devastation of this daily type of headache cannot be overemphasized. Frequently, the patient is depressed and desperate by the time the condition is recognized, as well as totally unable to withstand detoxification on an outpatient basis. Often, it will be the patient himself who recognizes the situation and subsequently seeks relevant therapy.

For the patient who is suffering severe headaches and is not able to function professionally or socially, and in whom depression has become a factor, hospitalization is recommended. It should be noted that this syndrome can develop with even fairly small amounts of aspirin or acetaminophen of no more than 1000 to 1500 mg per day.

TREATMENT

While most patients initially resist the idea of hospitalization for something as "trivial" as a headache, they frequently can be convinced of the necessity for this based on their degree of disability. Several studies have disagreed concerning the effectiveness of hospitalization, but many studies have validated this as a long-term solution for over half the patients who complete the therapy.

The goals of the therapy are fairly simple. The medications must be completely withdrawn as soon as possible and the various symptoms of the withdrawal state should be treated as effectively as possible.

Of course, not all medications *can* be safely withdrawn abruptly, including ergotamine, butalbital, and the various narcotics.

What happens during this withdrawal experience? The initial forty-eight hours are generally unpleasant for the patient. Many times, the patient experiences symptoms of an extremely bad migrainous attack. The nausea may be overwhelming, and the patient may experience vomiting to the point of dehydration and severe chemical imbalances. For this reason, intravenous feeding (IV) is frequently given during the first forty-eight hours.

The nausea is often controlled with anti-emetics such as prochlorperazine (Compazine) or metoclopramide (Reglan). Intravenous DHE 45 and methysergide have also proven quite helpful in this context.

After the first forty-eight hours, the patient will begin to recover, and a new course of treatment can be planned—one which does not rely solely on the medications that ultimately made the patient sicker.

Psychotherapy will often play a role in rehabilitating these patients, although it should be remembered that these patients did not begin using medications to achieve some sort of euphoric "high." Instead, they began taking the medications to relieve their headaches or their fear of these headaches. Depression, psychological trauma, and other psychological factors can of course influence the patient's analgesic abuse and should be dealt with appropriately.

Does Withdrawal Work?

Not all physicians agree that this regimen is effective, but studies do indicate a good response. Silverstein and Silverstein (1992) have reported that 87% of the patients completing detoxification remain free of analgesic abuse at a two-year follow-up after their release from hospital care.

DIFFERENTIAL DIAGNOSES:
SO WHAT ELSE COULD IT BE?

Below we will describe the more common and recognized headache syndromes. We must emphasize that a complete list of all types of headaches would be beyond the scope of this book.

Tension Headaches

Tension headaches, also called muscle contraction headaches, are the most common type of headache. Few people have escaped experiencing this problem at some point in life. As the name suggests, the tension headache is frequently associated with some type of psychological distress. The headaches are thought to be related to increased tension in the scalp muscles.

Most portions of the skull are covered with a layer of muscle. Contraction in these muscles leads to reduced blood flow and presumably results in the tension headache. Generally, there is tenderness about the cranium during these headaches.

The tension headache is frequently described as a "tight band" about the head or almost a "viselike" sensation. The headache may be a throbbing pain and sufferers may even report nausea and vomiting—some neurologists have said that this indicates there is a continuum between muscle contraction headaches and migraine headaches.

Although the psychological aspect of these headaches is emphasized, they can occur without severe psychological stress or underlying psychological issue.

There is no threat to life, nor is there any prolonged disability associated with the tension headache. It usually responds to medication. We educate our patients about the distinction between this and migraine, and often suggest proper body movements to avoid increased neck muscle stress and spasm. (See "Activities for Daily Living" in the Appendix.)

In addition, it is often helpful to do directed neck exercises (see "Neck Knowledge and Neck Exercises" in the Appendix) to reduce pain and increase flexibility and range of motion. This can frequently prevent exacerbations and future flare-ups.

Temporomandibular Joint Dysfunction (TMJ)

Only in the most recent decade have mainstream physicians accepted the TMJ syndrome as a problem that causes headaches. This resistance toward acknowledging TMJ as a headache cause may be due to the absence of abnormalities on diagnostic tests such as magnetic resonance imaging (MRI). Grinding or clenching of the teeth (bruxism) at night and gum chewing are often found with individuals who have TMJ. Generally, the pain is in the temporal region as well as the jaw area itself. An advanced TMJ syndrome can lead to severe difficulties in speaking and in chewing.

This type of headache syndrome responds well to splints, medication, and physical therapy. Severe TMJ syndromes can require surgeries, which, unfortunately, rarely succeed.

Neck Pain

We have found that head pain frequently is accompanied by neck pain that is often of a degenerative joint type (arthritic or disc disease). Although headache resulting from a neck disorder can occur without neck pain, this rarely happens; you usually get both.

The site of the pain is typically in the back of the head near the neck area. Tenderness is common. The joints of the neck spine often become inflamed, and these can act as a powerful pain source called a facet syndrome.

Sinusitis

The sinuses are located behind the nose at the base of the forehead and below the eye sockets. Infection in any of these areas will cause localized pain. Usually, there will be marked tenderness over the sinuses in the forehead or below the eye sockets. Post nasal drip (mucous collection in the throat when lying on the back) commonly accompanies this problem.

More advanced cases of sinusitis are usually associated with fever and a general sensation of being ill. If not treated properly, this condition can escalate and lead to infections of the brain or its covering membranes (meningitis, which we also describe in this chapter).

Sinusitis usually responds well to antibiotics although more resistant cases occasionally require surgical draining.

Trigeminal Neuralgia/ Tic Douloureux

Trigeminal neuralgia is a fairly common condition that primarily affects older individuals. The pain is of a shooting or lightning type. It generally last only a few seconds but can recur on a repetitive basis.

Frequently when some portion of the face or mouth is stimulated (a trigger zone), the pain is confined to one side and is usually below the eye, although the forehead can be affected as well.

This malady is caused by irritation of the nerve fibers near the base of the brain. Occasionally, tumors of this nerve or compressive lesions of the surrounding tissue cause this type of problem.

The pain is described as unbearable and can lead to total disruption of the sufferer's lifestyle. Fortunately, trigeminal neuralgia usually responds to the medication Tegretol, although occasionally it is necessary to destroy nerve fibers via a surgical procedure.

Occipital Neuralgia

This is a common disorder that is often missed by family practitioners and neurologists alike. Great controversy surrounds the frequency or even the existence of this disorder. We have found the condition associated with neck trauma in persons injured in automobile accidents. While the pain can be similar to the shooting discomfort of trigeminal neuralgia, it is typically more of an aching pain radiating into the eye socket. Often the person also feels nausea.

This condition typically responds to oral anti-inflammatory medications or local injections, although sometimes destruction of the nerve is necessary.

Eye Disease

We have rarely seen eye problems as a cause for headache, although certainly one exception would be glaucoma, in which the pressure of the eyeball suddenly increases. With this disorder, there is extreme pain in the eye and in the forehead, and vomiting may occur. Usually the white portion of the eye is very red. This condition is an emergency that must be dealt with by an ophthalmologist as soon as possible to avoid blindness.

Pseudotumor Cerebri

The brain and the spinal cord are surrounded by fluid that forms at the base of the brain and travels through various channels. Eventually this fluid is resorbed close to the large superficial veins near the inner portion of the skull. This fluid not only provides a hydrostatic "cushion," but it also is important to the nutritional status of the brain itself—a sort of brain food.

Generally, the pressure in the system remains fairly constant, but if the pressure of this cerebrospinal fluid is extremely high, then the blood flow to the brain will be stopped and death will occur rapidly.

Headaches can occur with cerebrospinal pressure that is too low or too high. Mild to moderate elevations of pressure inside the bony skull are seen in the condition known as pseudotumor cerebri. As the name implies, the clinical picture resembles that of a brain tumor, and in the past, exploratory surgery was performed on individuals presenting with this clinical picture.

The common symptoms are headaches occasionally associated with nausea and vague visual symptoms. This condition is more common in women, especially in women who are overweight. It may also be seen in people taking some medications such as antibiotics and vitamins.

Therapy involves medication and sometimes also requires a series of lumbar punctures or even surgery.

Cluster Headaches

The cluster headache is a fairly common headache, which is usually associated with pain in the forehead and eye area and generally lasts no more than an hour. The cluster head pain is often linked with watering of the eye on the same side as the pain, as well as with a runny nose. Sometimes the eye droops and the pupil on the painful side becomes small.

The patient may have several attacks on one day and these headaches may occur regularly. Individuals who suffer from regular cluster headaches may have very coarse skin about the face.

Cluster headaches respond fairly well to medication, particularly high-dose oxygen.

One variation of the cluster headache is chronic paroxysmal hemicrania. This type of headache is similar to cluster headaches, although it more frequently occurs in middle-aged women and usually lasts for 10 to 20 minutes. Such headaches may occur up to 12 times a day. Patients respond well to indomethacin (Indocin).

Temporal Arteritis (Giant Cell Arteritis)

Temporal arteritis, which primarily affects older individuals, is one of the more serious headaches and requires prompt evaluation and treatment.

The headache is usually described as a throbbing pain that is localized in the temporal area. Patients feel tired and ill, with an overall loss of energy. They may also report local tenderness, and merely brushing the hair may hurt. One frightening symptom is a sudden loss of vision in one eye. If this is neglected, vision can be severely impaired.

To diagnose this illness, a simple blood test, erythrocyte sedimentation rate (ESR) is often performed. This somewhat foreboding-sounding term refers merely to the rate at which red blood cells settle in a glass cylinder over a one-hour period. When giant cell arteritis is present, the ESR is usually several times the normal level.

In suspected cases of this disorder, an oral steroid is immediately prescribed, while preparations are made to remove a portion of the superficial temporal artery that is located in the temporal region. Prolonged therapy with oral steroids is often necessary.

Tumor

A common motivator for headache patients to see a doctor is the fear that they suffer from a malignant brain tumor. Yet only a very small minority of headache sufferers actually have brain tumors.

Headaches associated with brain tumors are fairly non-specific. If the pain is made worse by coughing, sneezing, or straining, or if it is generally worse in the morning, tumor would be a major consideration.

Meningitis

Severe headache is an almost invariable feature of meningitis. What is meningitis? It is an inflammation of the brain covering that results from infection. While there may be a history of exposure to meningitis or a history of middle ear or other infection, often there is no such history.

Viruses and bacteria account for most cases of meningitis, although many microorganisms can cause meningitis. Viral meningitis is usually self-limiting while bacterial meningitis is frequently fatal.

If diagnosed and treated early, the patient usually recovers entirely, although there may be such complications as seizures, deafness, or mental disabilities. The diagnosis of meningitis is confirmed with a spinal tap. (See the chapter on medical tests for further information on this procedure.)

Abnormal Blood Vessels

Various abnormalities of blood vessels can cause headaches. Arteriovenous malformations (AVMs) are abnormal blood vessels which channel blood from the arterial to the venous side of the circulation. Generally no headache results from this abnormality unless there is a hemorrhage. A hemorrhage can be life-threatening or it can cause fairly mild symptoms.

Headaches due to abnormal blood vessels may occur repeatedly, and for this reason can be misdiagnosed as migraine. Patients with this type of abnormality frequently have seizures, which complicate their clinical course.

Ruptured aneurysms also can cause severe headaches. An aneurysm is a "bleb" or a bubble-like expansion of an artery. The abnormal arterial expansion leads to weakness of the blood vessel wall and a high risk of hemorrhage.

The resulting condition, subarachnoid hemorrhage, is typically a sudden and very severe headache, often described by the patient as the "worst headache of my life." It is a true medical emergency and CT scan, angiography, and often lumbar puncture are needed to diagnose this condition. Surgery is usually recommended.

Stroke

Stroke can be defined as the death of a portion of the brain resulting from a disrupted supply of blood. This can be based on a clogged artery or a hemorrhage (excessive, sudden bleeding). The arteries are frequently blocked by debris from the heart or carotid arteries, or by the ultimate progression of atherosclerosis.

In the non-hemorrhagic stroke, headache is fairly common although usually mild. As with migraine, stroke frequently causes visual changes and thus can lead to a faulty diagnosis.

Medications

In a patient troubled by headaches, a careful medication history is essential. For example, it is now well known that aspirin as well as many other medications can actually cause headaches. In addition, suddenly withdrawing medications may lead to "rebound headaches."

Commonly used medications that are associated with headaches include nitroglycerin, captopril, indomethacin, cimetidine, and verapamil.

EMERGENCY HEADACHES

Certainly not every headache should lead you to rush off to your doctor. Some guidelines may help you determine when a medical investigation is a good idea.

A sudden change in the severity or type of headache, or the appearance of a new kind of headache in someone over the age of 50 should give rise to some concern. Also, headaches associated with mental symptoms or neurologic symptoms such as a drooping eye, muscle weakness, or the loss of balance should be reported to your doctor.

Headaches associated with intense neck pain or fever and headaches associated with straining, lifting, coughing, or sneezing suggest a more ominous type of headache. You should see your physician if your headache falls into these categories.

4

WOMEN AND MIGRAINE

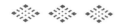

If you are a woman, your migraines may be triggered by reactions to food, stress, or any of the other causes discussed earlier in this book. Or, your migraines may be directly connected to the fact that you *are* a woman. Women do indeed have greater biologic basis to become migraine sufferers than men do, and female migraine sufferers are in fact more prevalent. Your migraines are more likely a combination of factors—such as eating a certain food (which may be a trigger), disrupting your normal routine sleep cycle, or experiencing severe stress or the onset of your period. Although any one factor might be enough to produce a migraine headache, in combination, they are almost certain to thrust you into a sick migraine.

Here we will discuss the prevalence of migraine headache disorder as it relates to women. In addition, we will discuss various aspects of your life that contribute to migraine susceptibility—self-esteem, family relationships, social activities, professional impact—and will expose a variety of misconceptions concerning migraine. Now known to be a true neu-robiological disorder, migraine headache pain can have a negative impact on many life areas if left untreated. In this chapter, we look at how the migraine spectrum changes throughout the course of a female's life, and point out a variety of specific techniques that can empower you to take charge of your headaches, even if you can't completely eliminate or control the biological factors that distinguish you from male sufferers.

FROM HORMONES TO HOT FLASHES

Over the last few years, we have learned quite a bit about the biologic basis of migraine disorder. Much credit should be given to the pharmaceutical companies for pioneering work in outlining distinctions and differences between female and male sufferers. Based on a variety of studies, we now know that the ratio of female to male sufferers of true migraine disorder is nearly 3:1. One in six females in the United States, approximately 18 million females, have at some time suffered a migraine headache. Interestingly, in a recent Princeton study of migraine headache sufferers, a majority of the women sufferers reported that they did not seek medical attention, as they did not want to be perceived as being weak, emotional, or "female." When questioned, they believed that others attributed migraines to emotional problems or stress, and they themselves did not see their headache as biologic in nature. When told that there was indeed a biologic basis for headache disorder, many migraine sufferers responded with relief; they felt reassured that they had a "legitimate disorder."

When the migraineurs were asked to relate why they thought women suffered 3:1 versus men, the vast majority of women believed that the difference resulted from environmental stressors, rather than from conditions involving hormones, biologic changes, or true physical changes. This lack of knowledge, understanding, and awareness of the basis of migraine disorder demonstrates that physicians need to improve communication with migraine sufferers, in order to outline the various treatment options that are available, rather than just telling patients to "try to get rid of the stress." Health-care intervention has improved a great deal, but your doctor is unlikely to take your migraine headache disorder seriously if he is unaware of its true causes.

SELF-ESTEEM

It is possible that the migraine sufferer experiences the most damaging impact in the self-esteem arena. Over one-third of the female migraine sufferers in the Princeton study felt that their lives were out of control, that they could not handle their migraines, and that this, unfortunately, further contributed to their inability to control their lives. This further demonstrates the need for awareness of migraine disorder, its triggers, and the variety of treatment options. Of the responders, over 80% described a sense of frustration, and over 40% of the female sufferers described feeling angry at their headache disorder. Over one-third of the sufferers felt resentment associated with the lack of control of their headache disorder. The same percentage felt resigned to accepting their migraine pain, suffering, and the downward spiral it typically exerted on their lives.

Another significant proportion—between 20% and 33%—felt either embarrassed or guilty over having migraine attacks, the guilt relating particularly to the effect that the migraine attack had on themselves, their family members, and their co-workers.

A patient of Dr. Kandel, Jane S., explained that her migraines had this effect: "I get up in the morning, and I don't know if I am going to have a migraine on that day. I start my breakfast, making sure to watch what I eat. For example, I have to avoid NutraSweet, as it has sometimes triggered attacks in the past. I get the children ready for school, then get myself ready for work. I am rushing all the time. In the back of my mind, I always worry: 'Will today be the day? Will I have to miss work? Will I have to call in sick? Will I have to go to the doctor?' It is a miserable existence, and I can't stand it. I just don't know when a migraine is going to hit me, and if it does hit me, whether I will be able to bounce back. What if I have to pick up my children at school? What if I have a play to attend? What if I have a major project to present? It just isn't fair. I feel like this thing has taken control of my life, and I can't get it back."

This frustration, resentment, anger, and guilt—particularly guilt for missing family outings—has had a negative impact on not only Jane S., but on many of our female migraine sufferers. Of course, missing a child's school performance or an important day of work obviously has negative consequences for the sufferer, but also affects the child or the employer. This then triggers a negative loop, which leads to the downward spiral of more frustration, more resentment, more anger, and more fear and loathing of the migraine headache.

One review study by the American Association for the Study of Headache revealed that discrete differences in mothers suffering from migraine headaches led to a negative impact on younger children. Migraine-suffering mothers of children under 12 would frequently have to find an alternative childcare provider, would miss more school activities, would not be able to attend projects, would not be able to participate on as frequent a basis with homework, and would have a great deal of guilt about being a "bad parent."

Furthermore, this study revealed similar results for mothers of children over 12 years of age, but for different reasons. Apparently, the older children were not able to engage in the same social activities as children whose parents did not have migraine. For example, they could not have friends over for fear that mother would have a migraine; would have to turn down their music, limit their activities, or not go out in a social sphere because "maybe mom won't be able to pick me up." Also, because of increased peer pressure, the stigma of having a mother with an "illness" was more likely to play a role. Again, the migraine sufferer experienced the same feelings, but mentioned them for a different reason.

In addition, women suffering from migraine were found to have impaired general medical health. Almost 50% of females with migraine stated that they consumed more prescription medicines because of the migraine headache disorder. They also had a deranged sleep cycle, which both aggravated and contributed to the migraine. One-third of responders felt that the migraine led to depression, and slightly more than one-third reported stomach upset, gastritis, or other gastrointestinal symptoms associated with migraine.

Migraine obviously has a significant bearing not only on how others see migraine sufferers, but also on how women with migraine see themselves.

FAMILY

In today's changing times, women play a variety of roles in the family unit—co-worker, parent, primary child-care provider, nurturer, and spouse. A variety of studies show that between 50% and 70% of females state that increasing stress in their life plays a significant role in their migraine headache disorder. That stress is attributed to the new roles women are expected to play. However, not all women who take on these multiple roles develop migraine disorders. It appears that women who have better coping skills have less frequent and less severe headaches than do those who lack the necessary coping skills. Also, those who have an appreciation for the degree of stress in their life seem to fare better; those unaware of the high degrees of stress are often unable to address or treat that stress, thereby triggering migraines.

In the women migraine sufferers surveyed, 90% explained that the higher stress they experienced was due to the combined child-care and increased household responsibilities. Two-thirds of these responders felt that their stress, which triggered migraines, was having a negative impact on the family as a whole.

As mentioned previously, women suffering with frequent or severe migraines experienced guilt, anxiety, and fear over their headaches. This played a significant role in how they reacted and responded to their children. A common thread in a number of studies was that female sufferers of migraine resented missing family activities.

Along the lines of family interactions and spousal relations, the stability of the marriage seemed to suffer due to the role that migraine attacks played. Over half the women surveyed explained that they would have to either cancel, postpone, or change activities based on their headache disorder. This lack of predictability, particularly when it led to canceling social activities "at the last minute," often played a negative role.

Linda B., who occupied a stressful position as secretary with a high-powered law firm, reported that she was always concerned whether she would be able to get her work activities done on time and avoid missing deadlines. A review of her headache diary revealed something she failed to notice: Immediately after completing a major project, or as soon as she had a few days off work, she would have a terrible migraine attack. Since she invariably planned major family events to follow the completion of her work, almost every family event had to be canceled. This upset Linda so much that she considered quitting her job, even though it provided a major income for the family. She eventually realized, by reviewing her headache journal, that work stressors were indeed playing a role, much more so than other factors in her life.

Changing her time to task completion, making workplace modifications, and explaining her headache disorder to her employer went a long way in reducing these severe "killer attacks," which she had previously experienced so frequently.

In addition, sexual intimacy is frequently impaired when it comes to migraine attacks. The expression "I have a headache" was never truer than when voiced by a migraineur. Not only does the headache pain, nausea, and a multitude of additional body symptoms make it virtually impossible to reach arousal, but the sense of inadequacy, decreased self-worth, lack of control, and negative self-esteem that result from migraine have an influence on your desire for intimacy with your partner. Communicating with your partner, particularly your awareness of the headache disorder, makes it easier to explain that it is difficult to be intimate. Also, involving your partner in the headache treatment, whether it be relaxation therapy, massage, meditation, or any of the other alternative interventions discussed in chapter 11, makes reaching a state of intimacy much easier, and often leads to more frequent and healthier sexual relations with your partner.

PROFESSIONAL

As mentioned above, migraine attacks commonly affect work activities—making a presentation in the boardroom, completing a job for your boss, or concentrating well enough to delegate responsibilities appropriate for your co-workers. The migraine headache can often rear its ugly head at absolutely the worst time.

A patient of Dr. Sudderth, a female executive, was noted to have severe sick migraines every time she was scheduled to give a boardroom presentation. She often had no choice but to turn this task over to her assistant, as she experienced severe intractable nausea. However, with the advent of Imitrex, she could excuse herself when she felt the prodrome, step to the bathroom, and give herself an injection (she always carried the injectable Imitrex). Within minutes, she would be back in the boardroom—bright, alert, and able to carry on. She barely missed a step.

While such boardroom heroics may not fit your lifestyle, as a woman who experiences migraines, you certainly face a number of barriers in the workplace. First of all, because they lack awareness, many co-workers and employers still see migraine as a "women's disorder" and view sufferers as weak or emotional, fitting the female stereotype. While this image is changing, unfortunately it is changing too slowly. Many employers lack understanding of migraine disorder, which may make the working environment even more stressful for the migraineur. As already mentioned, stress can act as a trigger; therefore, a difficult working environment may keep your migraine cycle going. Many sufferers feel that the combination of being a woman and a migraine sufferer is "a double whammy" that makes advancing in the work force virtually impossible. Women perceive employers as being more sympathetic to men who are ill, and believe that their employer views them as using migraine as an excuse to do poor or incomplete work (see Princeton study, page 38). Not only did many sufferers feel that their migraines had a negative impact on their work, but they also felt their employers did not provide appropriate accommodations to enable them to abort the migraine when it did come on. Being allowed to take breaks, make changes in workplace (such as go to a dark, quiet room or otherwise avoid light, loud noises, bright lights, heat or cold) often prevents the onset of a migraine.

We tell our patients that educating their employers before they are in the throes of a migraine attack can have a very positive impact. Specifically, we encourage them to explain that ten minutes of down time when they feel the threat of a migraine can help them avoid a full headache attack with the accompanying nausea, requiring time off from work. Workers who use flex time or a break to abort the headache often find they can easily make up that time later by working through a scheduled break. Having an employer who knows what your attacks are like and what to expect—in other words, taking the "fear" or mystery out of the attack—can do much toward improving workplace relations.

MISCONCEPTIONS

We know that female sufferers outnumber males 3:1. It is important to note that a true biologic/genetic component is responsible for this. Rather than dismissing migraine as a "female disorder," women must instead recognize it as a chemical/genetic/hormonal disorder that they can address as they do other medical conditions.

Why do women have such a high preponderance of migraine when compared to men? Is this always the case? Actually, in the pre-adolescent phase, girls suffer migraines at the same rate as boys, almost 1:1. However, with menarche (the onset of a young woman's menstrual cycle), the hormone surge begins and the ratio jumps to 3:1. Numerous studies have found a cyclical relationship of migraine headache disorder to the premenstrual or menstrual time of a woman's monthly cycle. Some patients experience the onset of their migraine two or three days prior to the beginning of menstruation. Other women tend to have migraines at the onset of menstruation or one or two days into the menstrual cycle. In both cases, the relationship of the hormonal changes to migraine attacks is clear. These migraine episodes have been given a specific name, "catamenial migraine," which means migraines related to the woman's menstrual cycle.

One researcher seems to feel that such migraines are related to the fluctuating levels of hormones, particularly estrogen, and the rapid rate of change, particularly dropping levels of estrogen. In addition, as with any physiologic function, other processes occur as well. Swelling, "bloating," and other physiologic processes may act as triggers. The psychologic stressors of menstruation may play a role, as well as the woman's overall general medical health. Some female sufferers who have particularly severe menstrual cycles, with cramping and other "PMS" symptoms, may also have a lower threshold for migraine attacks. As we have seen earlier, migraine episodes seem to be associated with additional medical problems. Menstrual cycles may actually play a role in lowering one's "illness threshold."

Several medications described in this book, such as Imitrex, have proven effective for women who suffer with migraines related to PMS and the hormone syndrome. Some physicians also recommend preventive treatment for migraineurs who suffer with catamenial migraines; for example, some recommend a percutaneous (through the skin) estradiol gel to stabilize the dropping rate of estrogen during the phase immediately before and during the menstrual period. Other physicians have found success with Propanol, a heart medicine that is also used for preventing migraine activities. Still others use abortive medicines, such as the anti-inflammatory Amitriptyline, when they believe their cycle will start.

In order to be able to take medicines two or three days prior to the onset of menstruation, the patient must be able to anticipate when her cycle will occur (in other words, be fairly regular).

In addition, as we have explained more than once, a migraine often has a multifactorial basis. Not only do existing stressors play a role, but chemical and food stressors have an effect as well. Avoiding activities that are known to trigger migraine makes good sense, especially at the onset of menstruation. In addition, avoiding common migraine triggers such as chocolate and caffeine is a good idea, no matter how much your body craves these substances.

Other triggers noted earlier in this book include stress, change in the weather, fluctuations in diet and skipping of meals, and bright light. Each of these triggers migraine for anywhere from 40% to 62% of the population. Reducing these environmental, internal, and external stressors at the time of menstruation can help you avoid the onset of a sick headache, or minimize the duration of a headache episode if it occurs.

What About Pregnancy?

Pregnancy is a peculiar time in a woman's life. The onset of pregnancy brings a true hormonal storm. Interestingly, after a number of hormonal changes occur, the estrogen levels seem to stabilize. Monthly migraines often abate, at least for the duration of the pregnancy. Unfortunately, other symptoms of pregnancy play an even more significant role. It is important to realize that migraine disorder in pregnancy may be especially difficult to treat, since avoiding medications in the first trimester is absolutely necessary. We suggest that all women who suffer from migraine discuss this with their obstetrician and develop an effective plan for migraine treatment prior to pregnancy. Many of the alternative therapies discussed in chapter 11 can help pregnant women eliminate the migraine or at least reduce its severity.

Labor and delivery is another stressful time, emotionally as well as physically. Even the positive emotional stress may act as a migraine trigger. As during the pregnancy state, medication management is essential, which means therapy options are limited. Additional considerations include whether or not the mother will breast-feed, as many medications used for migraine can be conveyed through the breast milk. Again, discussing this issue with your physician prior to making your decision is important. We had an unfortunate case of a woman who had status migrainosus (continuous migraines without abatement) after delivery. The physician and the patient were frustrated, and ultimately elected not to breast-feed in order to allow the mother to be treated for her headache disorder. If this had been anticipated prior to the labor and delivery, the woman might have tried any of a variety of alternative coping skills, relaxation strategies, or non-toxic medications. It is wise to discuss various plans with your physician, not only before becoming pregnant but also during pregnancy and before labor and delivery. If necessary, ask your physician to refer you to a good neurologist who has a particular interest in migraine headache disorders.

MENOPAUSE

A large number of baby boomer women (born 1946 to 1964) are heading into menopause. Many eagerly anticipate this life event, as menopause represents hope of relief from migraines.

Unfortunately, not all women experience pain relief during menopause. While many do obtain relief, the ratio of female to male sufferers drops only to 2:1. Menopausal women are still twice as likely to suffer from migraines as are men of a similar age. In addition, physicians often place their menopausal patients on hormone replacement—specifically estrogen pads, patches, injection, or tablets—for a variety of reasons, including cardiac disease and general medical wellness, but more often to avoid problems of osteoporosis (bone loss) and to treat other focused symptoms of menopause.

It is extremely important that you discuss with your physician whether or not you have had migraines in the past, and whether or not your hormone treatment, birth control pills, or estrogen therapy has ever been related to migraine attacks. Because birth control pills are indeed a form of estrogen, it is important that you explain to your physician what role your primary contraceptive regimen played in your migraine headaches.

Also, make sure you are truly in menopause before you agree to take estrogen. In one case, a woman's doctor decided that a 30-something woman was probably in early menopause because a variety of symptoms had presented. The patient had a subtotal hysterectomy in her late 20s, and believed that both her ovaries had been removed. Her doctor assumed this information was correct, and ultimately placed her on estrogen. Starting within a few months and continuing over the next few years, she experienced severe headache and fatigue, and finally realized that higher estrogen levels could be causing her migraines. She had a blood test done and found out that her hormone level was extremely high. She stopped taking estrogen, and as her level came down, her migraines went away. When her physician urged her to resume taking estrogen, her migraines came back. She ultimately stopped the estrogen and found a new physician.

The moral of this story is that if you are under age 50 and still have your ovaries (or might have your ovaries), insist that your physician run a simple blood test to determine your hormone levels before you agree to take estrogen. If your levels are abnormal or low normal, monitor your symptoms and look for alternative causes for your migraine symptoms.

MEDICATIONS CAUSING MIGRAINES

Medications can greatly influence migraines and migraine symptoms, as well as cause them to occur. For example, birth control pills can cause migraines, particularly when you first start taking them, as well as just after you stop taking them. As previously mentioned, changing levels of estrogen may trigger migraines.

Birth Control Pills

If you are on birth control pills and suffer from recurring migraines, you should consider an alternative method of contraception. The pill is certainly easy, efficient, and effective, while many other birth control methods are messy and annoying. However, the pill may be causing or contributing to your migraines which, as discussed previously, can dramatically affect sexual intimacy. Rather than changing your lifestyle or relationship, changing your hormone therapy and contraception is more likely to be effective. If choosing another form of contraception can abort or remove the trigger of your migraines, such a change is certainly worth considering.

Keep in mind that it may take three to six months to "clear" your system of birth control pills; don't expect to reach hormonal balance overnight. We tell our patients not to expect immediate pain relief.

Estrogen Replacement Therapy (ERT)

Estrogen replacement is often used in women who are suffering the early stages of menopause. Family physicians or gynecologists often place patients on estrogen therapy because it is an easy way to get rid of hot flashes (sweats) and other discomforts of menopause. Unfortunately, estrogen may also bring back or trigger dormant migraine disorders. However, a small percentage of migraine sufferers respond favorably to estrogen replacement therapy.

If you took the pill as a young woman and had to stop taking it because of migraines, hormone replacement therapy may once again act as a migraine trigger. However, this possibility should be discussed with your gynecologist. As we age, our basic physiologic functions change; and although you responded in a certain way earlier in life, hormone therapy may produce a completely different result at this point. Also, changing the dosage, frequency, and brand of estrogen replacement therapy may have a very positive impact on your frequency and severity of headache activity. Explore all the options open to you, particularly as you try to balance one medical benefit (prevention of osteoporosis or reduction in menopausal symptoms, for example) to a completely different benefit (prevention of sick migraines).

MEDICATIONS THAT WORK

Many of the medications described earlier are extremely effective for women with catamenial migraines. For example, in one research trial, 669 menstruating women, all suffering from migraine, were found to experience significant pain relief with Sumatriptan, as compared to a placebo (sugar pill). Indeed, this medicine appeared to work even better in women who had true menstrual migraines compared to those who had migraines not related to their menstrual cycle. Also, the Sumatriptan medication appeared to provide significant relief for up to 24 hours.

Many other medications have been reviewed and discussed in relation to migraine therapy. Some medications that are specifically effective for the migraine associated with menstruation include directions that they be used during the first few days of menses. Such "water pills" not only can reduce the headache pain, but can also reduce bloating and other physiologic problems associated with menstruation. As would be expected, water pills are most effective for women who suffer from excessive water retention.

Alternatively, recent studies show that many of the "tryptan" medications are extremely helpful, not only for migraines in general (for both men and women), but for women who suffer migraines associated with the menstrual cycle. In our practice, we are studying the role of Amerge, a long-acting tryptan, and its effect on catamenial migraine. We often start patients on Amerge two days prior to the menses, and continue throughout the first two days of the menses. Because initial results have been very positive, we feel this therapy merits further investigation.

As you can see, migraines can certainly behave differently in the two sexes. However, only women endure cataclysmic hormonal changes that act to confound the headache pain syndrome. The onset of menstruation, contraception, pregnancy, labor and delivery, and ultimately menopause are all confounding factors that play a role in migraine disorder. Physicians can help patients avoid treatment failures by listening to the patient, taking a careful history, and potentially by reviewing a migraine headache journal (a record of symptoms, triggers, and response to treatments) that the patient may be able to provide.

THE COMMUNICATION CONNECTION

We have established the importance of appropriate headache pain management after an accurate diagnosis is made. However, both depend on the patient being an active participant in his or her health care. To improve your diagnosis, enhance your headache pain management, get appropriate treatment, and gain the satisfaction of being a partner in your own health care, follow these steps:

- *Obtain help:* To get the appropriate diagnosis or the appropriate treatment, preferably seek attention from a licensed practitioner who has a special and keen interest in migraine management. Be a self-advocate; be comfortable explaining your symptom complex, and describing what helps and what doesn't.

- *Educate yourself:* It is important to learn as much as you can about your migraine disorder. The better informed you are, the more clearly and concisely you can explain your symptoms to your physician, and the more likely your physician will be able to make the appropriate diagnosis.

- *Make the appointment specifically for your problem:* We repeatedly hear from our family practitioner and general practitioner colleagues that patients visit their offices for a multitude of complaints, but rarely for their symptoms of headache/migraine. It is almost an embarrassment for patients to point out that they are there to discuss their migraine disorder. As neurologists, headache pain specialists, we see less of this reluctance to discuss the migraine issue. By the time patients come to us, many have already tried and failed to communicate their symptom complex at appointments with other physicians.

- *Provide a careful history:* We stress the importance of patients providing accurate information. When the headaches occurred, their severity and frequency, any triggers, and any prior treatment (medications, dosage, and length of trial) is information critical to making the right diagnosis. It surprises us that many people have "amnesia" concerning the various treatment regimens they have tried. It is vital that we obtain this information in an appropriate fashion. The simplest way our patients can provide such information is by recording details of their migraine disorder in the "headache journal" we provide for them. The journal enables them to keep a careful and concise record of headache triggers, various therapies that have (or have not) provided pain relief. The better prepared patients are when they come in to discuss their migraine headaches, the more likely that their headache problem will be addressed appropriately.

- *Have realistic expectations:* Patients who have had a constant daily headache for the last 30 years sometimes expect to have headache relief within a day after their first office visit. That is unrealistic, if not impossible. We explain to patients with periodic migraine disorders that the migraine is a chemical/biological disorder; like diabetes, it can be modified but cannot be removed or cured. We are honest with our patients regarding what they can expect, and likewise expect them to be honest with us. Knowing what is going on in their lives and what acts as migraine triggers can help us reach an appropriate end point that focuses on reducing migraine frequency and decreasing the intensity of their migraines; it also increases our patients' coping skills.

- *"The devil is in the details":* We specifically provide patients with a list of detailed information, including a migraine headache journal, a migraine headache diet, things to avoid, things to practice, and a variety of techniques to be practiced in step-wise fashion (see chapter 11, "Complementary and Alternative Approaches to Migraine Pain Management"). As Dr. Kandel explains to many of his patients, "When I started out in practice, I naively told patients, 'You've got to get rid of stress.' Stress, however, is part of life. More realistically, we can learn to understand, accept, and deal with our inevitable stress. That strategy can make all the difference. Now, rather than telling patients they've got to remove stress, I provide coping mechanisms, adaptive intervention, and techniques that help patients truly cope with their stressful situations. Without specifics, even the most carefully laid out plan is doomed.

- *Be a good patient by helping your doctor be a good doctor:* In part, this means listening to the doctor and providing appropriate responses to questions. For example, if you will not or cannot participate in certain activities or interventions, tell your physician. If he or she is competent, compassionate, and caring, your physician will try an alternative intervention (assuming there is one). No physician—not even the most kind, caring, or compassionate practitioner—will be able to provide appropriate information input and feedback if there is not a continuity of care. This means frequent follow-ups—perhaps in the form of telephone calls, fax reports, periodic visits, and correspondence with other treating physicians regarding her symptom complex.

We tell our patients that the more active they are in their care and treatment choices, the more successful their treatment regimen will be and the more satisfied they will be ultimately.

5

Migraine in Children and Adolescents

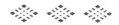

We have already discussed different headache types, particularly migraine, in adults. However, because children and young adults with migraine differ slightly from standard sufferers of migraine headache disorders, we will now focus on the younger age groups.

Medical History Is Critically Important

First of all, as in any good medical evaluation, the history is everything. One difficulty of treating children with migraine is obtaining a clear, concise, and accurate history. A child may not be able to describe his headaches and may not be able to characterize them or to explain their frequency, intensity, or severity.

In addition, a child may not have the language or the skills needed to describe the different components of the headache as most adults can. Therefore, it is crucial to have a clear history obtained not only from the child, but from other observers, particularly parents, siblings, and oftentimes teachers. Even school peers may add historical perspective, which can be extremely helpful in completing the puzzle that makes up pediatric and adolescent migraine.

Use a Headache Diary

As with other types of migraine and headache disorders, it is important to keep a headache diary, to determine if there are environmental, social, psychological, physical, chemical, or food triggers. (A headache diary sample is provided in the Appendix.)

Rule Out Serious Problems

Also, it is important to rule out serious or dangerous types of headache symptoms. Headaches that warrant immediate attention in the pediatric population would include the following:

- Headaches that are progressive in severity or intensity
- Headaches that are associated with weakness or clumsiness
- Headaches that are associated with a stiff neck or fever
- Any type of head tilt, head bob, or gait clumsiness
- A child with a chronic illness who develops headache
- Headache associated with a large head
- Children with chronic infections, particularly of the ears, teeth, or mouth

Categorize the Headache

Barring a serious organic or structural illness, headache disorders in children should be classified into either migraine type headaches or muscle type headaches.

While the characteristics are not absolute, frequently children suffering from a migraine headache disorder will describe a throbbing, hemicranial (one-half of the skull or head), periodic, sick headache.

In contrast, those children and young adults suffering from muscle contraction headaches will often describe a severe pulling, stretching, or tearing type pain, often at the base of the skull. Often, the child will describe the headache as being located everywhere over the scalp and head, not in just one isolated place.

The headaches that are muscle contraction in origin are often daily, chronic, and last for a significant period of time. There are rarely any associated neurologic, motor, or sensory deficits, or any associated nausea.

"Runs in the Family"

Children with migraine disorders will often have a strong family history of migraine, as do adult sufferers. The migraine may awaken the child from sleep, and may be associated with a warning or aura, as we described earlier with many adults. Muscle contraction headaches are often lacking these characteristics. In addition, children with migraine disorders often will respond to traditional migraine medications, while those with muscle contraction headaches will rarely respond to migraine medications.

Sleep Can Help

As we were taught during a neurology training program, and which has become an invaluable lesson throughout our practice, children who suffer from a migraine headache disorder often have "sick headaches." Frequently, the best therapy is sleep, and parents will often respond to the question "What makes the headache better?" with an unequivocal "Sleep!" If children experiencing migraines can just get to sleep, when they wake up, they're often fine.

Children also have an incomplete form of migraines, experiencing the nausea, the acute vomiting, and the extreme fatigue frequently associated in adults as the post-migraine chemical depletion. After a period of sleep, the neurochemicals of the brain seem to be restored, and the children have their routine energy once again.

Common or Classic?

Children with migraine can often have all forms of migraine, including common migraine without a warning or aura. They can also have "classic migraine," which often begins with the visual disturbance, described frequently as flashes of lights, zigzag lines, jagged lights, and patterns of light distortions.

Many times we find that instead of having children describe the pattern of lights and the disturbance to us, if we ask them to simply draw the pattern of disturbance, we can get clear and precise details with regard to their migraine warning.

Of possible concern is a child who presents with a complicated migraine. These children can have the full spectrum of migraine illness, as well as complications such as weakness, numbness, and clumsiness, which often mimic a stroke-like syndrome. Any time a child presents with a complicated migraine, neurologic evaluation is absolutely necessary.

Confusional States

We should make one brief comment regarding a variant of migraine headache—the headache disturbance that presents predominantly as a confusional state. Oftentimes, children with periodic confusional episodes will have a diagnosis of seizures, of daydreaming or staring spells, or of hypo-glycemia.

Actually, migraine can present in any form, and in young children, it does rarely present as a confusion and disorientation syndrome. However, we find that this is a diagnosis that is made only after other more serious diagnoses have been excluded. Diagnostic testing, such as MRI or CAT scan of the brain, brain wave scan, and often, lumbar puncture, is usually necessary to exclude other more serious illnesses.

Migraine with Seizure Disorder

In addition, a small percentage of individuals have migraines connected with seizure disorder. Children who suffer from migraine headaches often have abnormalities on the brain wave scan during the headache disorder, which then become normal between headache episodes.

It can be quite complicated to differentiate between a seizure event that is not accompanied by involuntary movements and a migraine headache disorder that is accompanied with altered blood flow in the brain, producing abnormal brain wave changes.

Other Symptoms

Although children may have the headache pain without associated symptoms, a majority will also have the nausea, vomiting, stomach cramping, and abdominal discomfort that adults often suffer when they experience migraine attacks.

Just as in migraines affecting adults, in a pediatric migraine, the stomach wall activity slows down during the acute migraine attack. For that reason, many medications are indeed ineffective. Therefore, often we must resort to using medications that are not given by mouth, but rather by rectal suppository or even by injection.

PRECIPITATING TRIGGERS FOR CHILDREN AND ADOLESCENTS

While we have described different types of headache symptoms in children in the previous paragraphs, it is important to realize that, in addition to the standard migraine triggers, there are many other precipitating factors in the child population.

Often, psychological factors, such as change in school environment, as well as physiological factors, including change in hormone level, onset of menarche, and dehydration, play a role in triggering migraines. Children are also extremely sensitive to fluctuations in routine, particularly to missed meals, as well as hypoglycemic events. This is a frequent cause of headache syndrome.

By asking children to chart their migraine attacks, we can often identify certain foods that act as triggers. It seems simple enough to eliminate these foods from the diet; however, as many parents know, gaining complete cooperation from a child or adolescent is often difficult. For this reason, making reasonable compromises with diet modifications is often best for migraine prevention.

Sleep Problems

If the patient suffers from headaches related to a disordered sleep cycle, such as insomnia, multiple awakenings from sleep at night, or terminal insomnia (waking up too early), we find that pharmacologic as well as non-prescription sleep aids are often effective.

We have had a great deal of success using small doses of Ambien, a relatively new sleep medication. Of course, body height and weight measurements are absolutely necessary to determine the safety of any prescription medication.

Nevertheless, we find that when we can readjust the sleep cycle, not only is it beneficial for the migraine management, it often seems to provide increased energy and alertness during the daytime, which produces a positive effect in school performance. This seems to have a snowball effect, producing positive self-esteem and ultimately leading into decreased stress, anxiety, and a reduction in headache frequency.

TREATMENTS

We try to avoid significant centrally acting medications in our practice, as these will often cause clouding of consciousness, confusion, and decreased memory and attention, which can negatively impact school performance.

Rather, as with the adult population, non-pharmacologic treatments are often pursued first. We have found biofeedback, guided imagery, and relaxation techniques helpful in allowing children to control their own headache syndrome. This, of course, works better with older children and adolescents.

Headaches can also be an outward manifestation or cry for attention, particularly with depressed children. Since lifestyle changes and self-image issues may be triggering the headaches, counseling or supportive therapy that leads to helping the child develop adequate and appropriate coping mechanisms is often more effective in reducing the headache severity and frequency in the long term, rather than medication management in the short-term.

On rare occasions, we do use antidepressant medication, not only for the antidepressant effect, but also for its effect on the central nervous system chemicals, as described in other chapters. Particularly, medications with amitriptyline, nortriptyline, and serotonin seem somewhat more effective compared to other medications for depression and relief of headache pain.

Medications

When we do use prescription medications, we try to target the type of headache, the nature of the headache with regard to daytime vs. nighttime, and the associated symptoms that occur with each headache episode. For example, the children who experience confusion, dizziness, disorientation, and have positive brain wave scans are often best treated with medications such as phenobarbital, rarely with Dilantin or Tegretol. All three of these medications are also quite effective as anti-seizure medication.

A common medication for headache therapy and pain relief is cyproheptadine (Periactin), given two to three times per day in one-half to one 4 mg tablet, depending on the child's age and body weight. A beta-blocker (Inderal), a cornerstone of migraine management, is also very helpful.

We usually delay prescribing this medication until the child shows us a series of headaches, particularly more than two in any one given month. This is used predominantly for prophylactic (preventive) management, and it is not quite as effective for management of the acute migraine attack.

True pain medications, as we have discussed earlier, such as combination medications (aspirin, phenacetin, codeine, fiorinal #3) are often helpful for pain management. The side effect of these medications is that they do cause drowsiness, as do some of the barbiturate medications, and therefore the child will need to rest, avoid exertional activity, and avoid activities which require focused concentration.

These types of medications are habit-forming and possibly addicting. Medication by rectum, such as Phenergan rectal suppositories, are often quite effective for the nausea, as well as for sedation, which can be an effective therapy in and of itself, as noted previously.

Other medication, such as Cafergot, can also be given by rectal suppository or by mouth. Again, if the headache has been present than 30 to 60 minutes, medications given by mouth often lose their effectiveness, and do not produce any of the desired effects—pain relief, sleep initiation, and muscle contraction relief.

Conclusion

It is important to realize that no one treatment fits every individual; therefore, obtaining the history of each child is absolutely essential. Maintaining a careful headache diary, avoiding food triggers, and identifying and eliminating external and social triggers are extremely important, possibly even more so than in the adult population.

If a child with recurrent headaches fails to improve with the previously listed measures, a consultation with a pediatric neurologist or neurologist specializing in headache management is often necessary to help fine-tune treatment regimens.

6

Non-Food
Migraine Triggers

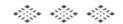

We've emphasized the critical importance of your physician taking a good headache history to enable effective treatment of your migraines. In the initial interview with you, as well as during your subsequent visits, the doctor must work hard to identify the primary factors leading to your headache problem. Once the identification of a trigger is made, you have an excellent chance of improvement with an effective, safe, and inexpensive therapy.

What's a Trigger?

A trigger is a factor, either internal or external, which can provoke a migraine attack. The trigger is not the cause of the headache, but acts instead as a catalyst that sets in motion the complex chain of events culminating in a migraine attack.

A trigger can be external stimuli, such as bright light, certain foods, or weather changes, to name just a few. Or a trigger could come from within, such as hunger, fatigue, or stress.

If trigger factors can be identified and subsequently avoided or minimized, then you will be saved from the prospect of medications or non-pharmacological treatments that could have side effects, cost big bucks, and have unpredictable effects.

More than half of all migraine sufferers will, with effort, be able to identify the trigger mechanism that is uniquely their own. But it is also true that susceptibility to triggers can vary even in the same person. For example, women may be more susceptible to triggers during the postmenstrual or premenstrual period than at other times during their menstrual cycle.

Age can also affect susceptibility to a trigger factor. Alcohol consumption is one good example of this phenomenon. Some people with a migrainous tendency are able to tolerate even large quantities of alcohol at a younger age, but later in life may find that even one drink of an alcoholic beverage can bring on an agonizing migraine attack.

It is also true that some triggers affect the sexes unequally. For example, one study revealed that weather changes, missing a meal, and the odor of perfume or cigarette smoke were much more common triggers of migraine in women than in men, while sexual activity seemed to trigger migraines more commonly in males.

COMMON TRIGGERS

Stress heads the list of all psychological triggers and also may be the most potent trigger of migraine in general. Some experts believe that more than 50% of all migraines are triggered by some type of emotionally stressful situation. And not only are migraines more frequent and severe during times of great stress, but the other bad news is that they tend to last for a longer period of time.

Many people who suffer from migraines identify the onset of the disorder in their lives as directly associated with a time of severe stress. Stress may be financial, academic, marital, or of some other nature.

In younger people, migraines triggered by stress may be associated with worrying about such things as examinations or plans to attend (or perform in) an important concert or recital. Sometimes the migraines that occur in these cases happen before the event and sometimes afterward.

Sometimes patients find their migraines cluster in weekends, which seems particularly unfair after a week of hard work. Possible reasons for this could be changes in sleep patterns, consumption of caffeine-containing beverages (more or less), alcohol use, smoking, or other factors.

Case History

A 45-year-old woman with a 20-year history of migraine was seen in our neurologic clinic. She was required to attend three to four major fashion events each year. Before each show, the patient experienced several weeks of intense activity related to preparing for the show. She sustained a very high level of activity until the end of the fashion show. Then, invariably, the patient developed a migraine attack that lasted three to four days.

Recognizing the stress of the fashion show planning as her trigger, we prescribed preventive medication as well as ergotamine, which proved ineffective in helping this patient. However, self-administered Imitrex has proven very effective in managing this woman's headaches, especially their intensity. Having access to rapid and effective treatment greatly increased her self-confidence as well.

Many Different Medications May Trigger Migraines

Sometimes a medication that you are taking to resolve another medical problem is your migraine trigger. Medications used to control high blood pressure, arthritis, estrogen replacement therapy (ERT), antibiotics, and even medications to relieve chest pain have all been implicated in causing headaches in susceptible people. In fact, many of these medications can cause headaches in people who are not usually prone to migraines.

Nitroglycerin is a good example of a medication that can trigger typical migraine headaches. While this medication can also cause headaches in non-migraineurs, it can lead to devastating migraines in susceptible people within minutes.

Indomethacin and other nonsteroidal/anti-inflammatory drugs (NSAIDS) can be effective in aiding the migraineur and can also cause an intense headache associated with an inflammatory response in the brain membranes. Withdrawal from this medication can cause an intense headache.

Illegal drugs are also associated with migraines. Heroin and cocaine use can cause headaches and migraines. Some people have become addicted to cocaine as a result of this drug's effect on the migraine. Such headaches can occur immediately after use or within the withdrawal phases.

Sleep

Many migraineurs report that inducing sleep is the most effective means of aborting a migraine attack, insisting that their migraine will not relent until they are allowed to sleep.

But besides being therapeutic in the treatment of migraine, an alteration in the sleeping pattern can be a potent migraine trigger in some people, possibly affecting women more than men.

Oversleeping can often cause migraine. So if you get up every day at 6:00 A.M., it's not such a great idea to sleep until noon on the weekend. In addition, shift work and jet lag should be avoided by susceptible people whenever possible. Of course, generating a "sleep debt," that is, going for long periods of time with less sleep than your body actually needs, may also be a powerful trigger.

Exercise

We frequently emphasize the value of exercise in this book because exercise can have a therapeutic effect on migraine. Yet it can also exacerbate a migraine attack, especially when the person is unaccustomed to a particular exercise. This problem seems to be more commonly associated with such intense activity as running and racquet sports, and tends to affect the sexes equally.

Many different factors that can contribute to the exercise-related migraine include climactic conditions and altitude as well as the hydration and nutritional state of the exercising person. Also, the changing heart rate, pulse, and breathing patterns associated with exercise can all play some role as migraine triggers.

Sexual Activity

Men whose migraines are triggered by sex find they occur near the point of orgasmic release. Such headaches are often indistinguishable from a typical migraine attack. Clearly such a headache can be very distressing. Not only that, but this kind of headache is often resistant to medications and thus can have devastating consequences for the individual.

Another sexually related headache is the benign sex headache, which, again, affects men more often than women. This type of headache also occurs right at the time of climax, but has no clear relationship to the migraine headache.

On the other hand, orgasm may also relieve the migraine in some people. One woman reported she was able to partially control her migraines through masturbation.

Smoking

Tobacco use can be a potent migraine trigger for some people. This appears to be more true for women than for men. There may be many reasons for this—tobacco increases carbon dioxide, decreases oxygen delivery to the brain, and actually acts as a direct toxin in some cases.

Hunger

Missing a meal can be a powerful migraine trigger in some migraineurs and also appears to be a problem more often for women than for men. In one study, missing a meal was a triggering mechanism in up to 40% of those suffering from migraine. It is possible that the mechanism for hunger as a trigger for migraine could be hypoglycemia, although there is little support in the literature for this theory.

Hypoglycemia can certainly cause migraines in some people and is often caused by the person eating a meal high in simple sugars. Shortly after eating such a meal, the blood sugar tends to rise, only to fall to a fairly low level several hours later. Avoid such meals if this is a problem for you.

Weather Changes

Many people report a migraine during a sudden change in barometric pressure, such as occurs prior to a thunderstorm. Women seem more susceptible to weather changes than are men. With drops in barometric pressure, joint capsules (such as in the jaw, hand/finger joints, and so on.) will swell. If there is any tendency for the joints to be inflamed (as in TMJ), this swelling will lead to pain and possibly trigger a migraine.

Sight and Sound

An estimated one-third of all migraine sufferers find that glaring sunlight is a triggering mechanism for their migraines, although how or why this happens is unclear. As a result, many migraineurs avoid exposure to bright sunlight, such as snow skiing, water outings, or trips to the beach or other situations. People with this problem may wear sunglasses virtually all the time that they are outdoors. Another related trigger is irregular illumination, such as fluorescent light bulbs, computer monitors, or strobe lights generate.

In some people, loud noises from heavy machinery, loud music, automobile horns, and such can trigger a migraine.

Odor

Certain smells can be strong trigger mechanisms for some people. This problem can be incapacitating when the sufferer is unable to eliminate these odors from the immediate environment. Odors that cause problems in susceptible individuals often emanate from gasoline and cleaning solutions, as well as perfumes, lotions, and deodorants.

Every effort should be made to identify the offending agent, and family members and others should be enlisted to help get rid of them. Individuals whose migraines are triggered by odors can be virtually powerless in many social settings.

Spinal Disorders

Over recent years, the medical profession has become increasingly aware of the tendency of spine disorders to trigger migraines. This is particularly true for neck disorders, but recent publications also suggest that back pain can contribute to headaches.

Osteoarthritis (the wear-and-tear arthritis) of the neck, as well as chronic muscle irritation related to injury or chronic tension, can trigger migraine attacks in susceptible people. In addition, neck injuries are often causes of increased frequency, duration, and severity of headaches in individuals who suffered from migraines prior to the accident.

In one study of patients with chronic low back pain, the researcher found that 60% of the patients also reported headaches. Only half of them had reported headaches prior to the onset of their low back pain. These headaches were not only muscle tension type but also migraine.

We have seen several individuals of both sexes in whom an exacerbation of the chronic low back syndrome was also accompanied by a severe attack of migraine headache. In the Appendix, we outline a series of neck exercises, as well as list many daily activities that, when performed properly, can help reduce these types of triggers.

Case History

A 28-year-old woman came to our neurologic clinic for evaluation of head and neck pain. The patient reported a ten-year history of migraines that were primarily left-sided and associated with photophobia, nausea, vomiting, and general malaise lasting up to 24 hours. Prior to a "whiplash injury" in a car accident, the patient had two to three headaches per year. After the accident, she reported daily headaches.

The patient was enrolled in a twelve-week cervical reconditioning program comprised of a rigorous daily stretching exercise as well as a biweekly strengthening program. During the course of the twelve-week regimen, the patient's neck pain improved, as did her daily headaches. The frequency of her migraine attacks has reverted to the pre-injury level.

ALLERGY AND MIGRAINE

The presumed connection between migraine and allergy is certainly not new. For over a hundred years, debate has raged on over what the actual role of allergic reaction is in producing a migraine headache.

While most neurologists do not feel that an allergic reaction is a potent migraine generator, the concept still has staunch advocates, including the support of public opinion. We hear at least several times a month from patients who are convinced that they suffer from migraines as a direct result of allergy. Part of this misconception is the patient's inaccurate definition of migraine. It is true, however, that allergies can certainly cause headaches. For that reason, we will discuss the nature of an allergic reaction and explore the basis for allergy as a legitimate trigger of migraine.

What Is an Allergic Reaction Anyway?

The word allergy is a composite of allos (other) and ergon (action), implying some type of mobilization against foreign chemicals. The "allergen" is the chemical toward which the allergic reaction is directed.

After an organism is exposed to an allergen (sensitized), then arsenals of chemicals (antibodies) can be produced by the body to react with the invading allergen. When the added allergen and the antibody unite, a kind of biological hell breaks out. Different types of cells are immediately summoned to the war zone. Potent chemicals are produced and released near the site of the first skirmish.

The result is essentially an inflammatory response with the attendant swelling, increased blood flow, heat production, and often, pain. If this reaction occurs in your nasal membranes (rhinitis), there will be increased production of secretions (runny nose), sneezing, and various degrees of narrowing of the nasal passages. If this occurs in your airways (asthma), the typical wheezing of the asthmatic is observed and some degree of narrowing of the air passages can occur. Occasionally this can be fatal.

It should also be noted that allergens do not have to be foreign substances, but can be part of your body; for example, some diseases cause the body to begin forming antibodies to its own tissues. An example of this would include some types of arthritis, lupus, and possibly even diabetes.

How Does Allergy Relate to Migraine?

Early (and continued) contentions that migraine and allergy were inevitably and inextricably connected were not based on any formal research but were merely the project of unschooled speculation. Now we do have some documented evidence of a weak link.

In the first half of this century, there were frequent reports of patients who were allergic to various foods. The reported patients had some type of allergic skin response to a specific type of food, but these claims were not substantiated by formal, case-controlled studies.

In addition, there was at least one report of a patient who developed a migraine when given a food type to which he had a demonstrated allergy. However, it was later demonstrated that when that same patient was not aware that he was consuming the alleged allergen, no headache would occur.

Another major problem with this type of research is that patients frequently will have a positive skin allergic response and have no type of demonstrable allergic symptoms and also no migraine. The more modern serologic studies aren't much better.

A fairly convincing evidence for a connection between food, allergy, and migraine was published in 1985. In this study, patients who had allergies to various foodstuffs, including wheat, corn, egg, and so on, were tested with food challenge (served a meal containing the suspected allergen). These patients were found to develop a headache within thirty minutes of ingesting the offending food item, even when they were unaware they had consumed it.

Some of these patients were demonstrated to have increased levels of histamine (an important chemical released during an immune response) in their blood after eating the food.

A more recently published study demonstrates correlation between food allergy and migraine. This study focused on children, age seven to eighteen, suffering from migraine. The children were divided into two groups: those who continued their customary diet, and those placed on a hypoallergenic regimen, which included only eight very simple foods for a duration of four weeks.

Members of the control group demonstrated no change in their headache pattern, while the diet-restricted individuals improved. Fifty percent of the diet-restricted group found their headaches were entirely eliminated, while most of the others reported a significant improvement in the pattern of the headaches. The most common offending food types in this study were cacao (chocolate), banana, egg, and hazelnuts.

The Histamine Connection

Histamine is discussed in this context because of its role in the mediation of the allergic response. Interestingly, histamine can cause dilation of the blood vessels in the scalp, which is seen in migraine, and can also cause severe, throbbing headaches, even in patients without migraine.

Typically, patients with migraine will get a headache from a smaller dose of histamine than is needed to generate a headache in a non-migraineur. In addition, the headache usually is experienced on the side where the migraine usually occurs. This so-called histamine headache can be entirely blocked by medications that block the effect of histamine, while these same medications have no effect whatsoever on a genuine migraine attack.

Some German authors believe that migraine is caused by histamine, but not on the basis of allergy. They feel that the histamine in the diet leads to a migraine attack. For this reason, they have proposed a regimen for elimination of histamine from the diet.

The investigators developed a diet in which fish, cheese, sausage, pickled cabbage, wine, and beer were excluded for four weeks. The authors report a major reduction in the frequency of headaches on the elimination diet. They furthermore postulate that the basic biochemical defect in the patient is actually a deficiency of the enzyme involved in the biochemical elimination of histamine. We find this an interesting theory, but certainly one that will need further investigation.

Other Types of Allergy in Migraine

Population studies have been attempted to demonstrate a link between migraine and atopic (allergic) diseases, such as hives, asthma, and rhinitis. Both migraine and these allergic illnesses frequently occur in the same individual. But studies have not been able to demonstrate a clearly increased frequency of these two disorders in specific individuals. However, one study reported in 1993 has suggested that there may be an increased association between allergic disorders and migraine in children.

The largest association was with rhinitis, and the authors report that rhinitis is particularly common in children whose mothers suffer from migraine. At this point, we feel there is much conflicting information with regard to the coexistence of these two disorders in the same patient and await a more definitive resolution of this matter.

Back in 1955, an interesting study demonstrated that migraine headaches can be a consequence of allergic illness. Twenty-eight patients were studied, all of whom had migraines, as well as rhinitis or asthma. The specific allergens to which the patient was known to be allergic were injected into the patient, thus reproducing the allergic symptoms. In most patients receiving the injections, a typical migraine occurred.

It should be emphasized that none of the patients developed the headache without the other symptoms of the allergic state. Interestingly, the aura (see chapter 1) was never described by any of these allergic migraineurs.

It should also be mentioned at this point that people with these types of allergic illnesses also have other problems that can increase the frequency of their headaches in general, and more specifically, their migraines. For example, these patients are often depressed and stressed because of their chronic illness.

It should be noted that medications to block the action of histamines—including steroids, decongestants, and theophylline—can also affect the frequency and severity of headaches in people who are prone to attacks. Also, typical sinus headaches are often seen in connection with these disorders.

By being aware of possible triggers, you and your doctor can engage in a broad, open-minded search for the offending factor. The ideal outcome of any encounter with your physician is to eliminate your problem without drugs, surgery, radiation, or other potentially hazardous therapy. With migraine, this is often possible.

7

FOOD FRIGHT

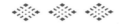

That migraines can be provoked by dietary influences is a fact that the lay public readily accepts. Many migraine sufferers have one or more foods they avoid.

The prospect of specifically identifying a chemical trigger in dietary migraine is a complex task. It should be remembered that triggers are facilitatory mechanisms that can lead to a full-blown migraine attack, only if various unknown other preconditions are met. For example, a long-awaited deadline may come and go without provoking a migraine attack in a woman whose menstrual cycle did not coincide with the deadline in question.

Similarly, a migraineur may imbibe large quantities of nitrite-containing foods or large amounts of red wine with relative impunity—unless the other factors involved in the migraine-producing process are also at work. Since response to a trigger varies even in a specific individual, it is difficult to research and form conclusions about this matter.

Furthermore, if a migraineur firmly believes that a specific food product will bring on a migraine attack, this is likely to occur as a self-fulfilling prophecy. Often, if the same patient is given the same food unknowingly, the migrainous response will not occur as predictably. Moreover, there may be a dose response for the triggering mechanism. Small amounts of the offending agents may be taken without provoking an attack. Even more perplexing is the fact that ingestion of the migraine-provoking agent may be related to a migraine attack already in progress, as is suggested with chocolate.

Food Triggers

Although much of the data presented in the literature on the subject of diet and migraine is anecdotal and based on questionable scientific rigor, we have concluded that there are potent triggers in the dietary sphere. As we have stated elsewhere in this work, the more systematic and open-minded the search for a trigger is, the more likely the individual is to succeed in identifying and eliminating migraine-provoking factors.

Alcohol

Alcohol is one of the most frequently identified dietary triggers by migraineurs. Interestingly, there is little documentation of alcohol per se as being the actual trigger. The studies to date suggest that the triggers are actually the various other components of alcoholic beverages that trigger a migraine in susceptible individuals.

Purer alcoholic beverages such as vodka, gin, and white wine seem to be tolerated fairly well by migraineurs while red wine is thought to be much more potent in terms of migraine stimulation. The chemical tyramine (vide infra) has been touted as being the offending agent in red wine. This has not been proven with any degree of certainty, but the observation that red wine is a more potent trigger is fairly commonly accepted.

Sugar Substitutes

Headache is a frequently reported side effect of the artificial sweetener aspartame (NutraSweet). This ingredient is used in diet sodas, as well as in a wide range of other products. The scientific data at hand are conflicting with regard to aspartame's role in provoking headaches. While this substance may not be a very frequent trigger of actual migraine headaches, it should be regarded as being suspect until further data exonerate this additive.

Caffeine

Caffeine is a ubiquitous substance in most countries of the world. It is abundant in coffee seeds and tea leaves, as well as in cocoa. In the American society, most caffeine is ingested through coffee drinking. Other sources would include tea, cocoa, and chocolate. Caffeine is also added to various over-the-counter pain relievers such as Anacin, and is also present in most soft drinks.

The role of caffeine in triggering migraine is probably not related to the immediate ingestion of this compound but rather to its withdrawal. Continued caffeine ingestion can be addictive, similar to nicotine, cocaine, heroin, and so on. The typical withdrawal picture includes headache, lassitude, restlessness, and even confusion.

Typical headaches undistinguished from typical migraine can be triggered by this withdrawal state in individuals suffering from migraine. Often, a cup of coffee will relieve headache symptoms. The withdrawal headaches usually occur by 16 hours after the last cup of coffee. It is not uncommon for the weekend to be a setting for caffeine withdrawal, as many individuals drink large amounts of caffeine during the work week and more modest amounts during the weekend.

Sodium Nitrite

Many preserved foods, including meat and fish, contain the preservative sodium nitrite. This substance, which is usually found in prepared meats such as bologna, sausage, hot dogs, and bacon, can cause severe throbbing headaches in individuals not suffering from migraine. They can also produce headaches undistinguished from a migraine in individuals suffering from this condition.

Many migraineurs avoid food products containing sodium nitrite since they can trigger headaches. It is the practice in our Headache Clinic to recommend avoidance of nitrite-containing products.

Citrus Fruits

Citrus fruits are universally touted as being among the most healthful features of any diet. However, citrus can be a potent trigger for migraines in susceptible individuals. It is thought that some of the nitrogen-containing substances in citrus have an effect on blood vessels and are capable of leading to a migraine attack.

While it would appear a bit extreme for migraineurs to avoid citrus altogether, careful analysis of the dietary diary should be undertaken to establish a possible role of citrus fruits in migraine provocation.

Monosodium Glutamate

Monosodium glutamate (MSG) is another chemical prevalent in Western diets. It is used as an additive to amplify the taste of various types of food. The consumer faces the difficult task of establishing the presence of MSG in many types of foods because euphemistic and confusing terms (such as "hydrolyzed protein" and "natural flavorings") are often used without specifically identifying the MSG content in a given product.

While MSG is inextricably associated in the popular mind with Chinese food, it is present in a wide range of food, including frozen dinners, potato chips, salad dressings, various seasoning products, and fast food such as fried chicken and hamburgers.

If MSG is ingested in sufficient amounts, it will produce a reaction that might include lightheadedness, abdominal pain, nausea, oral and facial numbness, headache, and chest pain within 30 minutes of the intake. This is popularly called the "Chinese restaurant syndrome."

Migraineurs frequently reported developing a typical migraine attack after eating even minute doses of MSG. It is the general practice of our Headache Clinic to advise patients to avoid foods containing this particular compound.

Tyramine

Tyramine belongs to a number of nitrogen-containing chemicals that directly or indirectly affect the caliber of blood vessels, thereby influencing blood pressure and the function of various organ systems. The effects of tyramine are similar to that of adrenaline and other related nitrogen-containing, physiologically active compounds.

After eating foods high in tyramine content, the migraineur may experience a typical attack within hours. The literature is rife with conflicting data regarding the importance of tyramine as a migraine trigger. In our view, it is a potent trigger in selected individuals, particularly if it is ingested in large amounts.

High tyramine-containing foodstuffs would include aged cheeses such as Brie, Roquefort, and Camembert. Many processed meats including bologna and salami contain large amounts of tyramine, as do sauerkraut and some beverages, such as beer and various wines. Migraineurs should be aware that many other foods have low levels of tyramine until spoilage. Improperly stored fish and liver can accumulate large amounts of tyramine over a fairly short period of time.

While the actual prevalence of tyramine-sensitive migraineurs is unclear, we recommend that patients in our Headache Clinic avoid large amounts of tyramine and we deliver instructions for elimination of these foodstuffs.

Other nitrogen-containing compounds with similar effects would include phenylethylamine, which may be the primary trigger in those individuals sensitive to chocolate. We think that there is good evidence supporting the concept of dietary factors as potent triggers for migraines in selected individuals. And yet we also believe that the influence placed on dietary migraine by many physicians, including some neurologists, is excessive.

Instead, we believe that a systematic approach—that is, a consistent and accurate dietary diary—is a more rational approach to dietary modification and will obviate indiscriminate banning of potentially nutritious and pleasurable classes of foodstuffs, rendering the migraineur a "dietary invalid."

DIET AND HEADACHE

According to the National Headache Foundation, the following foods may trigger migraine headaches:

Food that has been fermented, marinated, or pickled

Foods containing MSG

Sausage, bologna, pepperoni, salami, summer sausage, hot dogs

Chicken livers, paté

Herring, pickled or dried

Ripened cheeses such as Cheddar, Emmentaler, Stilton, Brie, Camembert (Permissible cheese includes

American cheese, cottage cheese, cream cheese, and Velveeta.)

Sour cream (more than ½ cup per day)

Nuts, peanut butter

Sourdough bread

Crackers or breads containing either cheese or chocolate

Broad beans, lima beans, fava beans, and snow peas

Figs, raisins, papayas, avocados, red plums (more than ½ cup per day)

Citrus fruits (more than ½ cup per day)

Bananas (more than ½ per day)

Chocolate

Pizza

Tea, coffee, or cola (more than 2 cups per day)

Alcoholic beverages (If you decide to drink, limit to two normal-sized drinks of Haute Sauterne, Riesling, Seagram's VO, or Cutty Sark.)

8

Choosing the Right Doctor

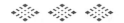

In your quest for diagnosis and treatment of your migraines, you need to find the best physician possible. So how do you do that?

Although there are many ways to find a physician who treats migraines, we think the place to start is with a qualified neurologist. So how do you find him or her?

Often, one has only to look in the phone book under the heading of "physicians" to find a neurologist—although we do *not* recommend randomly selecting your doctor from the phone book listings. The number of physicians available for you to choose from also varies depending on where you live. For example, in most larger cities, several neurologists practice in the given area, whereas in less populated areas there may be no neurologists for hundreds of miles. We think that at least your initial visit or two should be with a neurologist. Then, if geography makes frequent visits impractical, the local family practitioner can be the designated treating physician.

If you already have a family practitioner or internist, then certainly this question should be put to your doctor: Who is a good neurologist? Probably your doctor will also know a good neurologist with some interest in migraine (not all neurologists are intrigued by migraines). If a referral of this nature is not possible, then obtaining the name from a friend who is seeing a neurologist and is satisfied with the care would be another good referral possibility.

Occasionally there will be a neurologist in your area who has published work on migraine that you can examine in order to determine if this physician is right for you. Also, hospitals frequently have hotlines or printed material on specialists such as neurologists, but we urge caution here because hospitals often promote physicians who support the hospital's interest. Those interests may or may not coincide with yours.

A visit with a neurologist will not be inexpensive. However, the reason for the visit should be held in sharp focus. The cost of visiting the physician should be compared to lost wages and direct suffering related to the headache, as well as the suffering endured by the entire family when one member is severely affected by an illness of this nature.

Approach your physician with an open mind, but if it becomes clear during the interview or the examination that this physician is "just not right" for you, then try again. Keep in mind that migraine is a chronic illness, thus it is desirable that your relationship with your physician will last for many years.

Frequently patients will go to a neurologist chosen by the gatekeeper of their HMO, stating: "I have no other choice." While we do not choose our parents, siblings, or children, we can choose our spouses, friends, and, in our opinion equally important, our physicians.

While it might be reasonable to see the neurologist in your HMO initially, one should clearly have no compulsion to continue with that physician if a good patient-doctor climate is not achieved within one or two visits. Paying the neurologist's fee out of your own pocket when outside the HMO will often pay for itself many times over by saving you from pain, thus giving you more time for work and other pursuits.

So how do we go about making the right match? What is it about one physician as compared to another that makes him or her a good physician or, more importantly, the right physician for you?

Let's explain with an illustration. We perform many free educational seminars on back pain, neck pain, and migraine disorders, which we start with the sub-theme that open communication between the patient and doctor is essential.

One popular slide we use at our seminars pictures a golfer standing in a sand trap, looking up and asking a friend for a sand wedge. His friend hands down a sandwich to the baffled golfer.

If you find yourself constantly asking your physician for a sand wedge yet you continue to receive a sandwich, there is a lack of communication between you and your doctor.

SOME SIMPLE GUIDELINES

To get the most from each encounter with your physician, we suggest several guidelines:

- Be prepared. Know what your problem is or what your concerns are. Write them down. Bring any x-rays, medications, information on past medical interventions, and any information you have on your headache history. How old were you when they started? How severe was the first episode? How many headaches are you having per month or week? What seems to work? What doesn't?

- Ask the doctor if he or she is comfortable treating acute and chronic migraineurs. Not everyone is. For

example, some doctors state "I don't give out narcotics" as a pat response to pain management.

- Ask the doctor about how many migraine patients
  he or she treats in a year. Some doctors are not very
  experienced in treating this disorder and may provide
  elaborate explanations and little practical advice.

- Ask the doctor if he or she treats migraines with a
  variety of medications. If the doctor is resistant to
  trying new medications, this may be the wrong
  physician for you.

We often compare the doctor-patient relationship to a marriage, with the physician's office as the bedroom. Specifically, it
is an intimate place, where very important questions and
actions are undertaken, and frank, open, and honest discus-
sions regarding specific needs take place.

You need to be willing to share information and to be a
partner in your own health care. Be honest about what you can
and cannot do when it comes to treating your pain syndrome.

For example, one patient has assured us for four years
now that she will immediately discontinue smoking if "You
can just get me through this headache." But she has continued to use tobacco, which is a notorious trigger for headache
disorders. I've explained many times that this habit may be
playing a role in her migraine suffering, but this patient is
comfortable with a "quick fix" and is not interested in resolving the underlying problem.

On the other hand, some people just cannot remove certain triggers or life stressors. It's important to be honest with
your doctor about that as well. For example, if you have a difficult boss and a stressful work environment, and you have no
way of leaving your work station to abort an acute migraine,
tell your doctor. It does you no good if a treatment plan is
carefully outlined when you know there's no chance you can
follow it. Tell your physicians that you can't comply and ask
for another option.

Doctors Are Human!

It's also a good idea to remember that your doctor is a person, not a god. Still, the physician does not like to be challenged in a mean or nasty way, such as "Doctor, don't you know the latest information on that?" or "Doctor, I just saw 60 Minutes. I think that medicine will kill me!"

Instead, an assertive and positive statement such as, "Doctor, I understand there may be some side effects to this. Can you explain them to me?" or "Doctor, I'm concerned about some information I saw on TV last night regarding the medication you just prescribed. Can you explain why you want to use it? What are the side effects, and what can I expect?"

In a spirit of cooperation, mountains can be moved and migraines can be removed—if you work together with your doctor.

Evaluating a Prospective Physician for Yourself

What else constitutes a good match?

- Punctuality may be an indicator. If you are notoriously late and the doctor you see is notoriously on time, or vice-versa, then this may not be a good match.

- See how the staff treats you. *If* the first question out of a staff person's mouth is "How are you going to pay for this?" you may assume that money is the key issue here.

On the other hand, if the physician's staff asks for information in a pleasant way—for example, requests prior records, x-rays, documents, and so forth—you can be at least somewhat reassured that this doctor's primary concern is to get as much information as possible to come up with the correct diagnosis for you.

- Of course, your doctor's visit *will* cost you some money, and if there are particular financial needs that you have, it's a good idea to ask about the office financial policy on the first visit. Questions such as "Is there an installment policy?" or "Does the doctor bill the insurance company directly?" or "About how much can I expect the office visit to cost?" are all reasonable and appropriate to ask.

Sometimes you may have been referred to the new doctor by a friend, preferably someone with a similar problem who has done well with the physician you're planning to see. But do keep in mind that personalities are all different, and what one person likes in a doctor, another person may dislike intensely.

The bottom line is that you need to feel comfortable with the doctor and have confidence that he or she understands your problem and will listen to your complaints and try to do something about them. Do keep in mind, however, that if you've already seen twenty-five doctors, it is almost certain that there will be nothing magical about Doctor Number 26.

Health care is a precious resource and needs to be investigated thoroughly by prospective patients. You would not buy a new car (we hope!) without doing at least a little research. Nor should you trust your health to any doctor without doing a background check, office inspection, and even an initial evaluation to determine if this is going to be a positive experience.

Keep in mind that migraine pain is miserable enough without having to battle uphill with a physician.

9

Your Neurological Exam and Tests Your Doctor May Order

It's a good idea to have some advance knowledge of what medical information and documentation your new doctor will probably want you to bring with you to your first neurological exam, what kinds of questions he or she is likely to ask, and what types of tests your physician may order.

What to Bring to the Exam

When you visit your neurologist for the first time, besides bringing with you a positive attitude, you should be sure to bring medical records from other physicians who have treated you for other problems, including problems which don't seem to relate to your headaches or migraines.

Why? Because records that you may regard as irrelevant and unimportant may actually be very valuable to the physician who will try to help you with your migraines. And if the doctor does not need the information, that's okay too. It's better to bring "too much" than too little.

Important note: Plan ahead. Be sure to give yourself enough time to obtain those records. Call your other doctor(s) at least a week ahead of time whenever possible and find out when you may pick up the information and who can give it to you (that's usually whoever is in charge of medical records or the x-ray department).

Explain to the staff that the neurologist you were referred to is asking for complete medical records.

Keep in mind that sometimes doctors' offices do not like to release information directly to patients and consequently may insist on sending your records straight to the neurologist. The problem with this is that sending out medical records to Doctor B may be a low priority to Doctor A's staff—so low that they forget to do it.

If the staff absolutely refuses to release your records to you—and appealing directly to the doctor (their boss) doesn't help, then politely ask the staff when the records will be mailed. Be sure to call the neurologist's office before your appointment to make sure they actually received your records. (As a last resort, provide your new physician's fax number—you would be surprised by how many faxed records we receive on patients the day of their visits.)

Records that you *must* bring are your x-rays and MRIs. These are very important to the neurologist. Bring actual MRI films or CAT scans instead of written radiological reports because most neurologists are skilled at reading CAT scans as well as MRIs and may find abnormalities not observed by radiologists.

Cooperate as Much as Possible

Not to overstate the case, but remember to hold onto your positive mental attitude. Keep in mind that the doctor's goal is to empower you; and as you begin the diagnostic process with the physician, the responsibility for a satisfactory outcome is shared. Your good health care must be perceived as a joint doctor-patient goal. Think of yourself as providing evidence that your doctor will interpret, Sherlock Holmes–like, as clues to your diagnosis.

The initial phase of the "investigation" will consist of the clinical history. As is common with many other chronic problems, migraine is often diagnosed, at least in part, with the use of a questionnaire. (See the appendix for an example of a commonly used headache questionnaire.)

Certainly a questionnaire does not take the place of an intelligent doctor-patient dialog. The neurologist would much rather explore the nature of your complaints and precise responses (the best you can give) to the questions than hear a self-diagnosis. In other words, telling your doctor "I'm here because I have migraine" is not particularly helpful.

Even patients who suffer from migraines do not have their diagnosis stamped indelibly on their foreheads. Physicians must consider hundreds of possible conditions that could be causing the headaches. Failure to identify a serious, treatable cause of headache because you withheld requested information could be catastrophic for you.

QUESTIONS NEUROLOGISTS ASK

The physician will ask you when your symptoms started, how frequent they are, how long they last (minutes, hours, days?), and how severe they are. The doctor also needs to know about associated symptoms preceding, accompanying, or following the actual attacks. As has been mentioned elsewhere in this book, the diagnosis of migraine is based more on the recognition of a pattern of symptoms rather than on any one specific symptom or physical finding.

What medications are you now taking?   Lists of your medications as well as their effects on the migraine and their side effects will be of great interest to your physician. You might actually bring the medications in to show the doctor, so he or she can check the exact dosage, timing, and so on.

Are you affected by external factors that seem to trigger your migraines? Trigger factors are of particular interest. These may include habits such as smoking, or drinking alcohol or caffeinated beverages, as well as patterns of sleep, work, and sexual activity. (See chapter 6 on non-food migraine triggers.)

What is your emotional state? Your general emotional state, as well as the emotional state you experience during migraine attacks will be of interest to a skilled neurologist. Normal nervousness is okay, and the doctor knows that.

What is your medical history? This will be explored in great detail, to help in diagnosing as well as in deciding what medication you should be treated with.

For example, doctors will not prescribe the medication Inderal for patients with asthma. Patients with severe coronary artery disease would not be candidates for ergotamine or some of the other therapies frequently used in migraine treatment. Why not? Because these medications can lead to reduced blood flow to the heart or irregularities of the heart rate that would be dangerous for people with such illnesses.

Your physician is also likely to explore your family history (including your parents', siblings', possibly your children's) at length. Since relevant data are often not uncovered during the first visit (despite the best intentions of both patient and neurologist), the doctor will update your history at subsequent visits.

Be open with your physician, and don't be offended by questions related to tobacco, alcohol, street drugs, sexually transmitted disease, or sexual habits. The doctor needs this information to provide you with an accurate diagnosis and the best possible care.

The important thing to remember is that your medical history and your responses to the doctor's questions are the basis for making an accurate diagnosis of migraine. Although tests may confirm the findings or provide additional helpful information, we can't overestimate the value of a thorough medical history in diagnosing your condition and getting you on the path to improved health.

The Physical Exam

After completion of the history, the physician will begin the examination. We prefer to examine patients in a partially unclothed state. A gown is provided to the patient prior to the physical examination.

Initially, the neurologist will examine the cranium for evidence of local disease such as sinusitis, or tender scalp or arteries. The jaw joints are examined as are the eyes and eardrums. A brief examination of the teeth, mouth, throat, and so on is also performed. The physician is likely to examine various portions of the cranium as well as the neck and heart with a stethoscope. We also look for any abnormalities of the skin.

The Neurological Physical Exam

After a general physical examination, the physician will conduct the formal neurologic examination. This will include obtaining some idea of the patient's emotional state, intelligence, verbal skills, and thought organization. Simple tests of memory, abstraction, and more complex use of language are frequently given to supplement the mental status examination. You're not being given an "IQ" test so don't worry about giving the "wrong" answer. Just answer honestly.

Next the physician will undertake the cranial nerve examination to assess sensation in your face, movement of your face and tongue, as well as your sight and hearing. He or she will examine the retina of your eye with a device called an ophthalmoscope. Motor strength and coordination are tested as are the reflexes, the ability to perceive vibration, and other tactile stimuli. Don't be surprised if the doctor tells you to walk around the room or even in the hallway, since it's important to examine how you walk.

The Next Step for the Doctor

What happens next will depend on a number of factors. In cases in which the patient has a long, well-documented history of a benign headache condition such as migraine and has already had relevant testing including CT or MRI of the brain, no additional studies may be considered. However, in most cases of chronic headaches, the treating physician will usually order further tests. Generally, some blood tests and an MRI will be ordered, although other tests may be indicated too.

NEUROLOGICAL TESTS

There is some controversy about the necessity of tests in patients with garden variety migraine and who present a normal neurological examination. If your neurologist decides further testing is needed, often he or she will order imaging studies such as MRI or CAT scan of the brain. Since further tests may be indicated, we'll talk about those as well.

CAT Scans

The CAT scan (sometimes referred to by doctors as the "CT" scan) is a painless special kind of x-ray. Until the arrival and general acceptance of MRI scans, the CAT scan was the "gold standard" of brain imaging. Excellent views of the cranium and its contents can be obtained with this advanced technology. Hemorrhages, strokes, tumors, and increased intercranial pressure are frequently suggested by the CAT scans. In a patient with migraine, however, the CAT scans are generally normal.

Magnetic Resonance Imaging (MRI)

The MRI has proved to be a virtual revolution in medical diagnosis, particularly in relation to diagnosis of disorders of the brain and spine. When an imaging study is indicated in a patient with migraine, we favor this study because of its superior resolution and greater flexibility over CAT scans.

Please note: If you have had an MRI in the past, that doesn't necessarily mean you don't need another one. For example, your previous MRI may have been done years ago, or it may have been for a part of the body other than the head.

This type of technology is excellent for demonstrating stroke, most hemorrhages, and tumors, and frequently MRIs can actually reveal areas with subtle reduced blood flow—a common finding in the MRIs of patients with migraine. Abnormal blood vessels, which are frequently not seen on a CAT scan, often show up with excellent resolution on an MRI.

Intravenous dye material (don't worry, it's safe!), which provides better image contrast between abnormalities and normal brain tissue, is frequently given intravenously prior to completion of the study. More often than not, MRIs in patients with uncomplicated migraine are entirely normal.

What is an MRI like? The patient is enclosed in a chamber-like machine for this painless test. For the majority of patients, it's no big deal. However, some individuals experience claustrophobia-like symptoms—often people who never knew they were claustrophobic—and need to be medicated ahead of time with Valium or some other calming sedative. In some cases, patients are disturbed by the droning noise of the machine.

In our experience, from 15% to 20% of patients need some type of sedation when undergoing the MRI test. There does seem to be a technological trend toward less-enclosed MRI scanners; however, at present, we do not believe they are widely available. Our experience to date has been that the quality of the scan is not as good with these newer devices; however, advances in technology should rectify this problem.

With all its many advantages, however, the MRI will tell us little about inflammation in blood vessels and infectious processes, both of which frequently have headache as a prominent symptom.

The MRI is the most costly of the tests described in this chapter and can run about $1,200 or more.

Electrically Based Tests

Prior to the advent of advanced diagnostic imaging studies such as CAT scans and MRI, electrophysiologic (electric) tests were routinely used on patients with headaches. While this type of examination frequently turns up some useful data, it is still a crude technology when directed to the task of investigating structural lesions of the brain.

The electroencephalogram (EEG), the most commonly used electrophysiologic study of the brain, can be abnormal during a migraine attack. In this test, electrodes are placed on the scalp and brain wave patterns are measured by a machine. This is a painless test, and often patients fall asleep during the testing process. There is also a 24-hour EEG test, in which the patient carries around a portable machine, but such a test is almost never used by neurologists to evaluate headaches.

Usually the EEG between migraine attacks is normal; however, there may be some subtle changes. For example, certain features of migraine can be quite bizarre and are often suggestive of some type of epileptic phenomenon. The EEG is quite helpful in this regard. Abnormal EEGs are extremely common during an actual migraine attack.

Visual Evoked Potentials

This test has been available for about thirty years, although many lay people have probably never heard of it. It is not used frequently but may be indicated if a patient reports visual changes or has an atypical history.

Visual evoked potentials is a complex electrophysiologic test that allows the physician to test how fast and how well an image is transmitted from the eye to the portion of the brain involved with seeing (the occipital region). Sometimes injury to the optic pathways can cause visual complaints, and this test allows the physician to measure several different potentials.

During this test, the patient looks at a checkerboard that changes in some way, such as from black to white. Electrodes on the head will record the "potential" or impulse at various sites.

Certain abnormalities in this test are seen on a fairly frequent basis in patients with migraine. However, it must be emphasized that a normal or abnormal visual evoked potential does not with certainty confirm or rule out the diagnosis of migraine.

Angiography

Angiography is a test that allows indirect examination of blood vessels. This can be used for the head, neck, or other portions of the body. As a general rule, this test is not recommended for patients with a normal CAT scan or MRI. However, it can be important if there is some suggestion by history, physical examination, or (on the MRI) of some type of abnormal blood vessel, usually an AVM (arterial venous malformation), which is an abnormal connection between the arterial and venous blood supplies.

The angiogram involves some type of arterial puncture, usually in the groin area. A tiny tube is inserted up through the artery that leads into the aorta of the heart and then into the blood vessels of the brain. Dye is inserted through the tube to provide better contrast to show up in x-rays. Then x-rays in multiple planes are obtained, giving a three-dimensional indication of the size, location, and often the nature of the vessel in question. This test can be somewhat painful, although many patients report that it's not much worse than a blood test. The average test can take up to an hour.

Frequently the walls of abnormal blood vessels are thin and easily ruptured, which can lead to headache or even a stroke or severe neurologic dysfunction and possibly death. That is why advance diagnosis of such a condition is so important. The angiogram can provide this crucial information.

More recently, MRA (magnetic resonance angiography) has become available. It is not clear at this point if this type of procedure will replace conventional angiography described previously.

There has been some suggestion in the literature in the past that angiography in migraineurs carries an increased risk of injury to the brain. This risk has been borne out by definitive studies.

Thermography

Many physicians consider a thermography examination to be primarily punitive. Usually the patient is asked to disrobe and put on a skimpy garment much like a thong bikini. The patient is placed before a heat-sensitive camera during three sessions in which the emission of heat from various portions of the body is measured. About 60% of all migraineurs have a "cold patch" on their bodies between attacks. A cold patch is a small, well-demarcated area of reduced heat emission.

While results of this study are frequently abnormal during a migraine attack, the absolute diagnostic significance of the test is still far from clear. As a result, we rarely order this test. We note it here as a possible test that your physician may order.

Lumbar Puncture

Lumbar puncture (spinal tap) is rarely a reasonable measure in the diagnosis of migraine. In the spinal tap, the fluid (cerebrospinal fluid) that surrounds the brain and spinal cord is withdrawn with a needle placed in the lower back area. This test can be mildly painful, although a competent physician should be able to perform the test with minimal pain to the patient.

Chemical and microscopic examination of the fluid is often quite helpful for a diagnosis of diseases related to the brain. For example, many types of infection present very characteristic abnormalities in the composition of the cerebrospinal fluid. The content and composition of this fluid is normal between and usually even during migraine attacks. However, it is not unusual for abnormal cells to be found in the cerebrospinal fluid of patients suffering from an acute migraine attack. This test usually serves to exclude certain conditions from consideration such as hemorrhage, infection, or other inflammatory condition affecting the brain.

Laboratory Testing

If your doctor suspects there may be an inflammation of blood vessels of the brain, laboratory tests for arteritis or vasculitis, both inflammations of the blood vessels, can be ordered.

There are other laboratory studies which may also be helpful, such as tests to rule out thyroid dysfunction, anemia, diabetes, glucose abnormalities, and so forth. Your primary care physician has probably done a good general screening medical examination. However, if the neurological examination reveals specific deficits, such as loss of sensation, altered position, or vibration sense, then a B-12 level laboratory test may be ordered.

Conclusion

The most critical aspect of the diagnostic assessment is the patient history, and the most critical component of that history is the patient. Be as honest and accurate as you can. If you don't know an answer, it is all right to say so; but if you can, find the answer and report back later. Remember, this is not an inquisition, this is hopefully an establishment of a good ongoing relationship between you and your doctor—with the mutual goal of improving your health.

10

MEDICATIONS FOR MIGRAINE

"The desire to take medication is perhaps the greatest feature that separates man from animals." —*Sir William Osler*

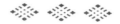

In this chapter, we will explore traditional medication management for migraine headache pain sufferers. There have been a number of recent breakthroughs in headache pain management. A variety of effective treatment regimens have evolved, and this chapter will explore them.

THE NOT SO GOOD OLD DAYS

When people in ancient civilization suffered from migraines, the "cure" was sometimes trepanning (drilling holes in the skull, often without any anesthesia), bloodletting after a careful placement of bloodsucking leeches, and/or dosing the patient with a wide variety of herbs, roots, and berries—generally foul-tasting concoctions. (Some people apparently believed that the worse the medicine tasted, the more effective it would be!) Ancient Babylonian priests created a mixture of burnt human bones mixed with cedar oil to rub on the migraineur's head, neck, and chest.

One treatment used in the first century A.D. involved the physician placing a hot iron against the forehead, which at the least distracted the person from the headache pain. Another treatment thought to be effective was pressing and rubbing the throbbing area with garlic.

Historical research reveals a wide variety of curealls for bodily ailments ranging from headaches to stomachaches to you-name-it. In the fourteenth and fifteenth centuries, for example, powdered Egyptian mummy dust was considered a very effective all-purpose medicinal treatment for whatever ailed you. Despite the fact that mummy dust didn't work (in fact, it made people vomit), European monarchs in particular favored it.

Throughout the ages people have used marijuana, cocaine, and other drugs that are now considered dangerous and illegal to alleviate suffering from virtually any illness. Alcoholic substances have been popular through the generations, as have been concoctions containing alcohol. Victorian women with "sick headaches" would have been shocked had they known they were imbibing alcohol—or perhaps they wouldn't have cared since migraine is definitely a leveler.

This chapter covers the lawful and effective medications we rely upon today to treat people experiencing acute attacks as well as recurrent migraines. Here you will find an overview of the broad array of the over-the-counter (OTC) and prescribed medicines—which ones work, their primary side effects, and important aspects to keep in mind about each medication. Keep in mind that if one medication does not work, another one or some combination of medications may be what you need.

In addition, the timing of medication can be important. If you wait too long—until you feel like your head is splitting open—it's often too late for many medications to work. That's because there is a significant time lapse between your getting the medication into your system and its being able to attack the problem.

The form of the medication is another major determinant in how well and how fast it works. Oral medication may take an hour or longer to take effect and the process is frequently complicated (as previously discussed) by your stomach functions slowing down during migraine attacks. An alternative route of administering oral medication is sublingual (under the tongue).

Intravenous injection (direct injection into a vein), subcutaneous injection (immediately under the skin), and nasal administration (inhaling) typically result in far more efficient delivery of the medication and have an effect within minutes.

Think of medication as soldiers fighting on your behalf. Send your "troops" into battle to assist you before you are too weak and debilitated to truly benefit! A far better strategy is to act when you feel a headache coming on by trying to prevent it or at least alleviate some of the pain. Of course, if for any reason you can't take the medication when you feel the migraine coming on, it's worthwhile to take something whenever you can. In addition, some medications (particularly those that are injectable) are very fast acting.

Another reason to treat the migraine as soon as possible is that a trip to the emergency room (ER) or a local hospital can often be a nightmarish, not to mention humiliating, experience. Why? Because ER doctors and nurses who are running around trying to help people with strokes, heart attacks, gunshot wounds, and other major trauma may be insensitive to the exquisite agony of the migraine headache. They may think, "Hey, it's 'just' a headache."

In addition, if you are viewed with somewhat jaundiced eyes in the ER, the staff is probably attempting to evaluate whether or not you are on the level. That's because a common ploy of drug abusers is to show up at the ER complaining of headache, insisting on a shot of Demerol or some other narcotic.

OVER-THE-COUNTER PAIN RELIEVERS

We have all heard of the most common pain relievers for migraine and other bodily ailments—acetaminophen (Tylenol), aspirin (Bayer, Excedrin), ibuprofen (Advil, Motrin), and most recently, naproxen sodium (Naproxen, Aleve). Indeed, some of these medications are also being clearly labeled as direct "migraine medication" to demonstrate to the public how effective they can be in migraine management.

These medications can help if they are taken early on in an attack and in sufficient dosage to be successful. Your doctor will base his or her recommendation on your medical history. For example, if you have a history of getting ulcers, your doctor will probably recommend you take the Tylenol and avoid the other over-the-counter medications discussed here. Why? Because the others can contribute to gastritis (irritation and inflammation of the stomach lining) and stomach ailments.

How much is enough? If you choose to take aspirin, an initial dose of 650 to 975 mg should be taken as soon as possible. Tylenol users should take 1,000 mg, which is equivalent of two "extra-strength" tablets. Keep in mind that because these are taken orally, the medication does not go directly from the mouth into the bloodstream and attack your pain problem. Instead, it must pass through the esophagus (food tube) and stomach to the small intestine (the site of absorption), and finally to the area needing pain relief. Peak blood levels (which indicate whether the medication is working at its best level) of aspirin and non-migrainous individuals is about two hours. But if the person is suffering from migraine, the medication action is slowed down considerably.

A common problem is that migraineurs may be vomiting so much that they lose all or most of the medication they have taken. You can combat this problem by supplementing your aspirin, acetaminophen, or other over-the-counter medication with an anti-nausea prescription medication known as metoclopramide (Reglan). Not only will this medication keep you from vomiting, but would also speed the transmission of the painkillers through your system. Reglan is most effective when given through intramuscular or intravenous injections.

Physicians can prescribe medications other than Reglan, of course, but many studies demonstrate that Reglan is quite effective in migraine headache management. One special protocol uses Reglan with an additional prescription medication to abort migraine symptoms. You may have to repeat this treatment a few times for maximum effectiveness because Reglan sometimes wears off before the migraine chemical change has completely resolved. However, knowing that medicines are available that can actually reduce the nausea and vomiting as well as relieve the overall suffering sometimes is enough to enable migraine sufferers to endure an acute attack. Certainly, knowing such treatment is available should reduce the anxiety many migraine sufferers experience with the onset of symptoms.

THE TRYPTAN REVOLUTION

Sumatriptan: The Miracle Medication

Sumatriptan (Imitrex), which is available in oral, subcutaneous, and nasal preparations, represents nothing short of a revolution in the treatment of acute migraine. The subcutaneous administration can stop a headache cold in dramatic manner since it gets in the system much faster than the oral preparation or the nasal spray, and patients can be taught to self-administer sumatriptan by injecting it directly under their skin.

One problem is that often the headache recurs within 24 hours. Side effects of this medication are usually benign: lightheadedness, flushing, weakness, and occasionally nausea and vomiting. Sometimes mild blood pressure increases occur. Patients over the age of 45 should receive an electrocardiogram (EKG) before having this medication prescribed.

Sumatriptan has been named even more than aspirin as a wonder drug of today. It not only can alleviate the migraine headache in 12 to 20 minutes, but can also reduce the uncomfortable side effects that often occur with migraine, such as the malaise of fatigue, confusion, and disorientation, as well as nausea and cramping of the stomach.

The pharmaceutical company that manufactures Imitrex has created an auto-injector that patients can carry discreetly. As a result, patients who are squeamish about giving themselves an actual injection can let the auto-injector do it for them without their having to view a needle. This medication comes in a discreet form that can be carried with the person without difficulty. By pressing the autoinjector against the skin and pushing a button on the unit, the medicine is automatically dispersed without the patient ever having to see a needle.

Before we allow patients to use this medication, we caution them to be forthright regarding their medical history—especially any history of chest pain or suspicion of coronary artery disease. Why? Because some narrowing of the heart arteries, or spasm of these arteries, has been reported with the use of the Imitrex injection. Despite this potential problem, we have found Imitrex an extremely effective medication that we have used safely in our office as well as in the hospital emergency room. We have seen no significant unfavorable reactions in our thousands of uses of Imitrex.

One young woman who works as an administrative assistant was extremely pleased with the introduction of Imitrex, which essentially changed her life. She had been averaging three to four migraines per month and required two to four days of disability time off each month. She was becoming very frustrated, as was her employer.

Now, she carries Imitrex injections in her purse, and when she feels a headache "coming on," leaves her office, goes to the ladies room, and gives herself an injection in the privacy of a stall. She stays there for about six to ten minutes then returns to her desk. No one knows that she ever had a sick headache! She recently informed us that she was promoted and credits the fact that she has had no more migraine-related absences from work. This enabled her to improve the quality of her work, as she has become a more comprehensive "team player." Her life is considerably happier.

Other tryptan medications have come along since the arrival of Imitrex, including zolmitriptan (Zomig), rizatriptan (Maxalt), and naratriptan (Amerge). These medications differ somewhat in their onset of action, duration of action, side-effect profile, and administration. All are available by convenient oral dosing, with Maxalt also available in a handy lingual wafer, which does not require fluid for swallowing. The wafer disintegrates on the surface of the tongue directly through the mucosal membrane of the mouth, which enables it to bypass the stomach ("your upset stomach"). This novel delivery with Maxalt has made it very popular with many headache patients.

Amerge, with which we have been having great success for the "rebound migraine," deserves some additional comments. Made by the company that produces Imitrex, Amerge is designed to be more effective for the longer-lasting migraines. We have been very impressed with Amerge's ability to alleviate the rebound migraine phenomenon. When patients respond to initial doses of Imitrex, Maxalt, or other medication, only to experience the migraine returning in four to eight hours, this is consistent with the migraine process outlasting the medication benefit.

Amerge has also demonstrated some success in alleviating analgesic rebound headache—that is, the headache associated with constant anti-inflammatory or pain medication management. A daily dose of Amerge, one tablet in the morning, for five days, can often be extremely effective in alleviating analgesic rebound pain. It can be helpful in breaking the cycle—by an as-yet unknown mechanism.

There will undoubtedly be more tryptans on the market in the near future. The "Tryptan Revolution" has truly lived up to its name and has altered anti-migraine therapy quite favorably.

Nonsteroidal Anti-Inflammatory Medications (NSAIDS)

The prototype of this important group of medications was aspirin and lower doses of over-the-counter medications such as Motrin, Aleve, and others that we have already mentioned.

Migraineurs may need larger doses (for example, as much as 750 to 1,000 mg of Naprosyn), which are available by prescription only. Medications frequently used in higher doses by physicians include ibuprofen (Motrin), diclofenac sodium (Voltaren), naproxen sodium (Naprosyn), ketorolac (Toradol), as well as many others.

We have had great success with a few anti-inflammatory medications, such as Voltaren, that can be given as a once-a-day dosing regimen. In addition, medications such as Arthrotec (an anti-inflammatory medicine combined with a stomach-protecting medicine) have also been extremely helpful. There are many classes of anti-inflammatory medicines, each of which acts from a slightly different chemical basis, as well as many medicines within each class. It's important that you understand which anti-inflammatory medication your doctor prescribes.

If a medication from one class doesn't work for you, you might switch to a different class of anti-inflammatory medication altogether rather than try other medicines in the first class. Medication use often confuses patients (and even physicians at times!). That is why patients should keep as accurate a diary as possible listing medicines that have worked or failed in the past. This record can ensure that a new physician does not have to start from "square one."

A new class of medication, "the Cox-II enzyme blockers," includes Celebrex and more recently Vioxx. These medications block an enzyme that prevents the inflammation from starting. Not only are they effective for osteoarthritis, rheumatoid arthritis, and for pain, but they can also be extremely effective in treating mixed muscle contraction headaches. Indeed, because of its significant effect on the joints, inflammation, and pain level, this new class has become one of the most rapidly growing medication types in this country. We have used these medications in combination with other medicines to achieve optimal pain control.

Midrin

Midrin is a compound medication that includes acetaminophen and dichloralphenazone, a general sedative. These medications are combined with isometheptene mucate, which helps constrict the blood vessels and reduce head pain.

We have used Midrin successfully for several years, and have seen numerous patients with fairly severe migraine greatly helped by this medication. Keep in mind, however, that "rebound headaches" (those caused by overuse of the medication itself) can occur if this medication is used more than two to three times per week.

It is also important to know that isometheptene mucate can be dangerous for patients who suffer from high blood pressure, liver or kidney disease, or glaucoma.

ANTIEMETICS (ANTINAUSEA MEDICATIONS)

Antiemetics are frequently invaluable in treating the acute attack because they enable the patient to keep the medication down so it can do its job. Also, since nausea and vomiting are sometimes the worst part of the illness for the patient, avoiding this aspect is quite a relief. Antiemetics include such medications as Reglan, Thorazine, Phenergan, Compazine, Tigan, and others that are available in oral and injectable forms, as well as in suppository form.

Side effects of antiemetics do occur, and the key ones are abnormal involuntary movements, reduced blood pressure, drowsiness, and anxiety. Sometimes, more serious problems occur such as liver disease, allergies, dermatitis (skin rashes), gastroenteritis, and even bone marrow suppression. Fortunately, the severe side effects are quite rare.

Ergotamine

A mainstay of the acute migraine attack, ergotamine, has proven effective for about half of all patients suffering from migraines. This medication can be administered rectally, orally, or by placing a tablet under the tongue (sublingually). Oral medications include Cafergot and Wigraine, which contain 1 mg of ergotamine and 100 mg of caffeine. Typically, two tablets are taken as early as possible during the headache and may be repeated every 30 minutes to a maximum of six tablets per day.

When discussing ergotamine (or ergot medications), one must remember that too much of even a good medication is not a positive treatment. We also want to carefully monitor the risks versus the benefits of any medication. And, as previously noted, individuals with other medical conditions can have problems taking this type of medication.

The rectal preparations of ergotamine, Cafergot suppositories and Wigraine suppositories, contain 2 mg of ergotamine and 100 mg of caffeine. One or one-and-a-half suppositories (depending on your doctor's direction) are inserted rectally at the onset of the headache and may be repeated after one hour. No more than two of these suppositories can be used per day. Our trick is to use one-half of a suppository at the headache onset rather than one full suppository. This can then be repeated every four to six hours for symptom relief.

Sublingual preparations of ergotamine include Ergomar and Ergostat, each of which contains 2 mg of ergotamine. Medications are placed under the tongue at the beginning of a headache and may be repeated every half hour for up to three tablets per day.

The ergots have a tendency to cause blood vessel constrictions. We found that when our patients use a dose high enough to produce any benefit or pain relief, both their veins and arteries are affected. It is important to monitor blood pressure, and to monitor the ultimate amount of ergotamine used. Patients with severe atherosclerosis, coronary artery disease, and high blood pressure should stay away from this medication. Also, we avoid using this medicine if the patient has a history of hypothyroid disease, or is currently pregnant or nursing.

The main side effect of ergotamine is nausea and vomiting, which can be relieved by prior administration of Reglan. Less frequent side effects are dizziness, muscle cramping, tingling, diarrhea, and abdominal cramping.

Dihydroergotamine (DHE)

Dihydroergotamine is a safe and effective medication that was until recently the unchallenged "gold standard" for the treatment of an established migraine attack. While chemically similar to ergotamine, it appears to be less constrictive of the blood vessels. In addition, unlike ergotamine, DHE is often very effective when the patient is in the throes of a severe attack. DHE is administered intravenously, intramuscularly, or nasally (Migrainal) for individuals who are squeamish about injections. This medication, often combined with Reglan, can be extremely effective in alleviating not only isolated migraine, but also cluster migraines.

Nausea is a common problem with DHE, and patients suffer the side effects of sedation, anxiety, diarrhea, and body aches. DHE is not recommended for patients with significant coronary disease, or poorly controlled hypertension. Pregnant women should avoid DHE.

STEROIDS

In severe, intractable migraine attacks, many physicians will use intravenous steroids. Often this will be after "tryptans," narcotics, and other measures have failed. Typically, we give dexamethasone (4 mg intravenous) after premedicating with intravenous Reglan. After the patient is able to tolerate oral medications, then we give another steroid, prednisone, for five to seven days. Although steroids have received generally bad press in recent times, we feel that short-term use of steroid medications is reasonable in the context of intractable migraine.

Case Vignette

Amy, a 30-year-old woman who suffers from quite severe migraines, was admitted through the emergency room because of intractable headaches, nausea, and inability to maintain hydration. She had recently undergone knee surgery, for which she had used narcotics to control her pain. Unfortunately, she had severe nausea, making it difficult for her to maintain oral hydration. Amy developed an intense, unilateral throbbing headache associated with severely intensified nausea and vomiting. When rectal antiemetic medications proved ineffective, she was admitted to the hospital where she was given a maximum dose of Demerol, Imitrex, and Reglan as well as IV hydration. She remained quite uncomfortable. The decision was made to administer 4 mg of dexamethasone intravenously, and within two hours her headache and nausea had subsided. At this point, she was able to leave the emergency room department.

Narcotics

Many physicians hesitate to prescribe narcotics for migraines, although most neurologists use this type of medication at some point in their careers. The problem is that studies show the risk of addiction for patients with migraine is high, and doctors do not want to add the problem of addiction to the recurrent migraines.

Narcotics prescribed by physicians for migraines usually include various compound formulations of aspirin or acetaminophen combined with propoxyphene, oxycodone, or some synthetic chemical. Samples of the proprietary medications of this type are Darvocet, Darvon, Percodan, Percocet, Vicodin, Lorcet, Oxy IR. Since these can provide rapid relief for patients who are in severe pain or are truly unable to tolerate other medications, they do act as an option, a temporary solution for the migraineur.

In addition, a commonly used narcotic is Tylenol with codeine, with variant dosages of codeine.

Tramadol (Ultram)

Tramadol (Ultram) is used increasingly for pain control of various types. A synthetic analogue of codeine, Tramadol has been compared favorably with meperidine (Demerol) for postoperative pain relief. It has also been used for dental pain as well as low back and other types of chronic pain, and appears to be as effective as acetaminophen with codeine.

There are sporadic reports of Ultram being effective in treating migraine as well as other types of headaches. Ultram seems to be more effective for mixed headaches, that is muscle contraction headaches combined with and/or triggering migraines. At this time, no well-controlled clinical studies establish tramadol as an effective treatment for migraine, although it does seem relatively effective for muscle contraction headaches. It appears to have very little abuse potential. Side effects include dizziness, nausea, dry mouth, and sedation, although these are relatively infrequent. Occasionally, isolated reports of seizure activity are associated with Ultram use. Pregnant women should avoid this medication.

Besides the oral medication already described, a very successful nasal spray is available. Stadol, often touted as a "rescue medication" for migraine sufferers, is convenient, safe, and frequently effective for acute attack of migraine.

Patients should be aware that continued, frequent use of the medication does pose risk. For this reason, physicians are loathe to use it indiscriminately. Nevertheless, Stadol is often a temporary solution for rapid relief for patients experiencing severe pain who are unable to tolerate other medications, or for whom other medications have been unsuccessful.

Stadol has proven effective in migraine, usually acting within 15 minutes. Approximately 43% of patients taking this medication complained of some somnolence (sleepiness), and many individuals report a mild sense of dysphoria (altered sense of self and mood). The convenience of this method of administration makes this a valuable tool for the treatment of an acute attack of migraine.

A common complaint is that our patients do not always know if they are really getting that first spray, and sometimes overdose themselves by taking a second inhalation in the other nostril, thinking that the first one "didn't get through."

We find that patients get excellent relief from their migraine pain, but can become relatively incapacitated if they are not cautious when using the medication. Often, educating patients on how to use the medication effectively and reminding them to follow instructions to "prime the pump" will alleviate this problem.

PREVENTIVE MEDICATIONS

If the patient suffers from recurrent migraines, physicians often prescribe a preventive medication. This decision is based on the severity and frequency of the headache, as well as on factors related to the patient's medical history and his or her ability to tolerate various medicines.

Many doctors recommend a prophylaxis (preventive) therapy for patients suffering from more than one attack a month; others suggest preventive treatment for those who have weekly attacks. Another guideline for determining therapy to prevent migraine headaches is the degree and severity of disability that occurs with these headaches. If your migraine headaches don't cost you much in terms of time or money, and are tolerated by those around you, then your physician may allow a greater number of occurrences per month before starting preventative therapy.

However, even one sick headache per month that produces significant disability, financial loss, or social complications may well indicate that it is time to try preventive treatment. Since there are no clear-cut guidelines, you should consult with your physician.

BETA-BLOCKERS

A class of medications that inhibit the effect of adrenaline and other similar compounds, beta-blockers affect the heart, blood vessels, lungs, and central nervous system. The most commonly used beta-blocker is propranolol (Inderal). If used properly, this medication can decrease the severity, duration, and frequency of the migraine attack.

This medication comes in various preparations, including a long-acting preparation. It is also frequently used for blood pressure control. Since it is used to treat patients with high blood pressure, as one would expect, a side effect could be lightheadedness, or low blood pressure. Indeed, a low pulse rate, and even airway constriction, can be a side effect. It is important to avoid this medication if the patient has underlying emphysema or asthma as a medical condition.

This medication may take three to four weeks before benefit is noted, so we encourage our patients to continue work with this medicine for at least two to three months. Also, dosage adjustments may need to be made to maximize the benefit of this particularly helpful medication.

As mentioned, if there is lung disease, you should consult your physician before starting beta-blocker therapy. Also, those individuals with severe coronary artery disease, heart rate irregularities, or lower extremity blood vessel problems should avoid this medication. Or, if additional medications are being used, such as ergotamine or blood vessel constrictors, beta-blockers would be contraindicated. Diabetics should avoid this medicine as well, as this can mask the side effects of a diabetic reaction, which may lead to significant problems.

CALCIUM CHANNEL BLOCKERS

Newer on the scene than the beta-blockers are the calcium channel blockers. These can be very effective for migraine prevention. They can decrease the frequency of headaches when the primary action appears to be on the blood vessels themselves. Side effects can include lightheadedness, flushing, even fainting. Medications including verapamil (Calan, Isoptin) is probably the most commonly prescribed, although some long acting calcium channel blockers (such as Covera HS) are quite effective. Nighttime dosage regimen can often be prophylactic for the migraine attack that can occur in the middle of the night. There are several calcium channel blockers available; and just like the beta-blockers, this medication class is used for heart disease as well.

It is not unusual to develop some mild ankle and leg swelling when using calcium channel blockers, particularly at moderate to high doses. While this is an annoying side effect, and one that can be alleviated with support stockings, it rarely limits the medication use. Like the beta-blockers, calcium channel blockers may not take effect for a series of weeks, and may require dosage adjustment.

ANTIDEPRESSANTS

Even if you don't suffer from clinical depression, you may benefit from taking one of the antidepressant medications described here. The reason for this is that these medications act on and cause changes in the brain that could alleviate the pain.

Prozac is in the class of serotonin-associated medications, and is actually a selective serotonin reuptake inhibitor (SSRI). As stated elsewhere, serotonin is a chemical messenger compound thought to play a role in migraine.

Prozac (fluoxetine) and other medications in this class are very potent and important therapeutic interventions. However, the negative press for writing Prozac prescriptions has made many physicians reluctant to prescribe this medication for migraine rather than for major depression alone.

Many migraine sufferers do experience clinical depression. This well-recognized association is addressed in several competing theories. For example, living with a chronic illness of any type has been shown to be a potent risk factor for depression. However, some theories suggest that migraine and the chronic daily headaches may deplete the pain-mediating neurotransmitter serotonin in significant neural populations (or possibly in some brain cells). This serotonin depletion may be a fundamental contributor to the development of depression. For these reasons, the antidepressant Prozac holds great promise for people suffering from migraine and depression, as its serotonin-depleting properties are, at least in theory, beneficial in both conditions.

Denise S. was a 25-year-old neurology resident who was greatly troubled by migraines, and had only mixed results with various treatments. Adding 20 mg of Prozac twice daily improved her headaches so much that she had only one or two fairly mild attacks per year. Initially, 20 mg of Prozac is used, although doses as high as 80 mg are sometimes needed. This medication is different from most other antidepressants in that there is little if any drowsiness; instead, an increase in energy is characteristic. Weight loss may occur. We recommend this medication not be taken close to bedtime, as its stimulant effect may lead to insomnia.

We believe that Prozac is one of the most important advances in the pharmacologic treatment of both depression and migraine in recent decades. The claims of the medication causing individuals to commit suicide are vastly overstated.

The other Prozac-like medications (SSRIs) include sertraline (Zoloft), fluvoxamine (Luvox), nefazodone (Serzone), and paroxetine (Paxil). There is little to suggest that these medications as a group are any more effective in terms of migraine prophylaxis than beta-blockers, tricyclic antidepressants, or Depakote. Of course, this is not to say that these medications may not be extremely effective in a particular individual. Anyone who treats patients with migraine should certainly keep SSRIs in mind.

Venlafaxine (Effexor) appears to represent a unique antidepressant. While this functions to a large degree as an SSRI (like Prozac), it also appears to affect pain-mediating pathways in the brain. For this reason, as pain specialists, we use this medication for many types of chronic pain. We have had excellent results with this medication for migraine prophylaxis. A recent Portuguese study demonstrated a favorable prophylactic effect in individuals suffering from migraine. The examiners did note side effects such as weight loss, nausea, and occasional vomiting. The researchers report a favorable prophylactic response in almost 90% of the patients. Venlafaxine is a potent but underused prophylactic agent in the treatment of migraine.

Traditional Antidepressants

Antidepressant medications have been around for years, and most of the older medications fall under the group of "tricyclic" or "heterocyclic," which are transformed to the chemical structure of these medicines. They have been used successfully for many years as a preventive treatment for migraineurs, and their effectiveness is clearly documented in the literature, especially for amitriptyline (Elavil, Endep) and doxepin (Sinequan, Atopen). They appear to influence all the major aspects of migraine headaches, including frequency, duration, and severity. Antidepressants may also be used in conjunction with other medications. For example, the combination of propranolol and amitriptyline appears to be particularly helpful.

Unfortunately, there are extensive lists of side effects associated with these traditional antidepressants. These include such things as dry mouth, lightheadedness, low blood pressure, cardiac rhythm changes, palpitations, drowsiness, and urinary dysfunction (difficulty starting the stream of urine, particularly for older men).

Additional medications in this class of treatment include Norpramin, Pamelor, Vivactil, Desyrel. These all cause similar side effects to a somewhat lesser extent. Often, these medications are prescribed at nighttime. This may make the side effect profile somewhat more tolerable, particularly the effect of extreme dry mouth and sedation.

The medications are usually started at low dose, and slowly titrated up to a therapeutic level. At the higher doses, many of these medicines can be monitored by blood evaluation. The effect on migraines may take four to six weeks to be measured, and a trial of two to three months is usually recommended. It is also recommended that an EKG be done on patients over age 50, or on any patients with prior cardiac history.

MONOAMINE OXIDASE INHIBITORS (MAO INHIBITORS)

Although we rarely use this class of medications, it is important to provide a complete list of possible treatments. MAO inhibitors should be used only if you are a person who will unconditionally follow your physician's instructions, and will report any side effects promptly.

Nardil is one common MAO inhibitor, and may be used alone or in combination with other traditional antidepressant medications such as Elavil.

The side effects of MAO inhibitors may be dramatic when they do occur. Side effects alone include occasional series alterations of behavior, abnormal involuntary movements such as tremor and muscle twitching, and even convulsion. Fatigue is very common, as is weight gain. Dryness of the mouth is another unpleasant side effect. Starting the stream of urine is often problematic, particularly in older men or individuals with prostate enlargement. Sexual dysfunction in both men and women is a common side effect.

Many medications must be avoided altogether when an MAO inhibitor is taken. This includes certain medications given for weight loss, asthma, and respiratory infections. The combination of these medicines with an MAO inhibitor could lead to serious side effects, including a severe uncontrolled high blood pressure. Use of illegal drugs, particularly cocaine, represents an extreme danger.

We urge extreme caution for our patients who use MAO inhibitors, particularly if there is any other "copharmacy" being utilized.

CYPROHEPTADINE (PERIACTIN)

Cyproheptadine (Periactin) does occasionally help for migraine prevention and can be an effective medication for prevention of migraine in children. This medication frequently causes drowsiness, dryness of the mouth, abdominal cramps, and urinary retention. Weight gain and increased growth in children have occasionally been seen.

An interesting case involved a nine-year-old child who was started on Periactin for his migraine disorder. There was a strong family history of migraine, with the patient's mother having difficulty controlling her own disorder. The child did well over a four- to six-week period of time, but gained about ten pounds and outgrew all his clothes. The mother thought her child was going through a growth spurt, but found it peculiar for him to gain so much weight in such a short period of time.

I discussed the side effects with the mother and child, and the child volunteered that he had a constant hunger. We switched the child to a different medication, and his headache disorder remained under good control. He dropped the ten pounds, and fortunately did not need an entirely new wardrobe.

TOPIRAMATE (TOPAMAX)

Topamax is relatively new on the market in the arena of pain management and headache prevention. This medication was originally designed and approved by the Food and Drug Administration as an adjunctive therapy for adults and pediatric patients for partial onset seizures. Recently, a number of studies have demonstrated the effectiveness of Topamax in the treatment of neuropathic pain. More recently, in the April *Journal of Neurology,* an article describes a potential role of Topamax in the treatment of intractable daily headache. The study seemed to reveal a decrease in the number of daily headaches; apparently, the improvement was significant. A number of theories have been postulated, although the exact mechanism of headache pain management is not entirely clear. Some of the actions include stabilizing the brain membranes and brain chemicals.

In our experience, Topamax has taken off as a very effective medication for the management of chronic migraine pain, for patients who have refractory migraines, and for those who have either rebound or cluster migraines. In addition, our female patients who have migraines associated with their menstrual cycle seem to respond quite well to Topamax, taken in a moderate dose three days prior to menstruation and the first two to three days during menstruation.

Clearly, additional trials and research studies will need to be performed, to determine the true level of effectiveness of this medication. However, for our patients who suffer from these refractory migraines, this medication has been extremely effective.

ANTI-SEIZURE MEDICATIONS

Valproic Acid

Valproic acid (Depakote) is relatively new in the treatment of migraine. In the past, this medication has been used primarily for various types of epileptic seizures.

Traditionally available in oral form only, valproic acid can cause liver dysfunction, especially in younger individuals. Therefore, this should be avoided in patients with a history of compromised liver function. It is often necessary to check blood levels periodically. Fairly common side effects of this medication are sedation, tremor, and loss of coordination. Other common side effects are loss of appetite, nausea, and vomiting. More uncommon side effects are allergy, hair loss, and weight gain.

A recent study in Denmark of 43 patients with migraine revealed that about 50% of the patients responded to this therapy. This seemed to affect predominantly the frequency of migraine, rather than the severity and duration of the patients' headaches.

In our practice, we have discovered that there may indeed be a dose relationship, in that a slightly higher dose of the Depakote medication may result in a significant improvement in headache prevention and control.

Recently, Depakote was approved by the Food and Drug Administration as an effective prophylactic agent for migraine management. In selected patients, this seems to be an extremely useful tool for migraine pain control. Recent reports suggest that valproic acid can be administered intravenously for abortive therapy of an acute migraine. Studies are underway to confirm these reports.

Other Medications

Other anti-seizure medications, such as phenytoin (Dilantin) and carbamazepine (Tegretol) are sometimes used in migraine prevention. In addition, gabapentin (Neurontin) has been extremely effective in chronic non-terminal pain management. It does play a role in certain individuals with migraine headaches.

Gabpentin (Neurontin) and topiramate (Topamax) have been reported effective as migraine prophylaxes. At the time of press, these reports are anecdotal and these medications have not been subjected to rigorous trial. However, physicians who are experienced in treating patients with refractory migraine may wish to consider these medications when other more commonly used prophylactic agents have failed.

CAN MY MEDICATIONS HARM ME?

Medication therapy is quite helpful in the treatment of migraine. In fact, the major advances related to migraine have been pharmacologic. In addition, most people who suffer from severe migraine attacks will at some point benefit from medication. However, certain medications over the long term can be harmful, can possibly cause migraines, and can certainly cause "analgesic rebound headaches."

Too Much of Anything Is Bad

Any medication can have side effects that can cause the patient discomfort, disability, and possibly death. For example, acetaminophen (Tylenol) has long been promoted as the ultimate in drug safety. However, as the studies described below indicate, even this over-the-counter medication can have serious side effects and should be used only as prescribed as infrequently as possible.

It has been known since the 1950s that pain-relieving medications can cause severe kidney damage. In fact, one medication, phenacetin, has clearly been shown to be responsible for kidney failure in many individuals using that medication. It was far less well known that the main metabolite (breakdown product) of Tylenol is phenacetin.

A recent study in the *New England Journal of Medicine* by Thomas V. Perneger and others gives some reason for alarm for those using a large amount of Tylenol. This powerful study provides fairly convincing statistical arguments discouraging use of this medication on a habitual basis. In this study, 716 patients with chronic renal (kidney) failure were interviewed and compared to 361 age-masked controls without kidney failure. Self-estimates of the amount of consumption of Tylenol, aspirin, and nonsteroidal anti-inflammatory medications were obtained. While there was no suggestion of increased incidence of kidney failure in those taking aspirin, there is evidence of hazards related to Tylenol and nonsteroidal anti-inflammatory medications. The studies suggest an increased risk of kidney failure for those taking up to 5,000 pills of nonsteroidal anti-inflammatory medication over the course of their lifetime. With regard to Tylenol, a daily consumption of more than one pill per day doubled the odds of chronic renal failure, as did a lifetime consumption of 1,000 pills or more.

It should be likewise noted that the risk of drug-related renal failure is increased in persons with diabetes or advanced age, as well as people with problems of dehydration— a frequent consequence of a migraine.

The authors of the study proceeded to make a dramatic suggestion: By reducing the overall consumption of acetaminophen in a population, the number of chronic renal failure cases might be lowered by 8% to 10%. They further suggested that the U.S. could save approximately $500 million to $700 million in estimated care for these patients with chronic renal failure.

We don't wish to single out acetaminophen, and recognize that patients who experience these side effects may have fared much worse on other medications. We use acetaminophen on a frequent basis in our patients. The point, however, is that we urge our patients to use it as directed and on an intermittent basis. We warn them that it can be very harmful to assume that any medication sold over the counter is automatically "safe."

At this point, we have potent and effective means for treating migraine. However, these therapeutic regimens often are a two-edged sword. Information we have included in this chapter should encourage migraineurs to rely as little as possible on medications for their treatment.

The following case illustrates how medication that routinely provides excellent pain relief may also play a role in producing a significant problem.

Complaint: Migraines

Gloria, a 33-year-old right-handed female, has a history of headaches associated with nausea, vomiting, and weight loss dating back to approximately age five. After two or three years (when she was age eight or nine), the headaches resolved until she was 26. She had seen three separate eye doctors, who attributed her headache pain to astigmatism. Gloria describes her headache as involving the whole head, associated with a "funny sound" in her ears as well as pressure around the skull. They were initially left-sided, but over a two-year evolution, began to involve the entire head. She has found that only emergency room visits for narcotics, sleep medication, and indeed the initiation of sleep are helpful for her pain.

Gloria has had an extensive list of medications, including anti-inflammatory medications, muscle relaxers, sleep medications, pain pills, and strong narcotics. Despite all this, she has continued to experience pain. She also sought psychiatric care, as she was concerned that there was a psychiatric component, although this has not been borne out. In addition, Gloria has seen neurologists and has undergone imaging of the brain on two separate occasions, and was told that these studies were normal. She has also had brain wave scans, again reported as normal.

Her history is complicated by irritable bowel, and by difficulty in tolerating medications. She has a history of mild asthma, kidney stones, and "blackouts" that occurred when she was pregnant. Gloria had been placed on numerous medications on a trial basis. Interestingly, she found that the medication Fioricet was quite helpful.

The history becomes interesting in that, without any type of narcotic abuse or excess, she ended up in the emergency room for drug intoxication. Unfortunately, she was labeled there as a "drug-seeking patient," and was given relatively quick attention. Gloria clearly was minimally responsive, lethargic, barely arousable. Her medication bottles were checked and she was not taking the medication any more frequently than two or three tablets per day.

She was admitted to the hospital, given intravenous fluids, and after two days, was much improved. Apparently, the erratic absorption of the Fioricet from her body fat tissues led to too much medication in her bloodstream and subsequently led to her unintentional drug intoxication or "overdose." This was a significant negative reaction to a medication that she was using as directed.

CONCLUSION

Your physician can try many types of medications. The key is for you to choose a good doctor with whom you can cooperate as a team to get rid of—or at least cut back on—the frequency and severity of your migraines. We hope that the information presented in this chapter will further motivate and educate patients to assume responsibility for their care.

11

COMPLEMENTARY AND ALTERNATIVE APPROACHES TO MIGRAINE PAIN MANAGEMENT

A Short History of Medicine:
"I Have a Headache . . . "

2000 B.C.	"Here, take this root."
A.D. 1000	"That root is heathen. Here, say this prayer."
A.D. 1850	"That prayer is superstition. Here, drink this potion."
A.D. 1940	"That potion is snake oil. Here, swallow this pill."
A.D. 1985	"That pill is ineffective. Here, take this antibiotic."
A.D. 2000	"That antibiotic is artificial. Here, eat this root." —*Anonymous*

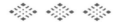

We have already discussed many aspects regarding migraine care in this book. We covered the basics of migraine headache disorder, the different types of headache syndromes, and a variety of mechanisms that are presumed to cause migraine headaches. We have also talked about the explosion of new medications as well as more traditional medication interventions for the treatment of migraine headache pain. In addition, we have looked at various subgroups of migraine disorder, as well as described a variety of migraine triggers for individual sufferers. However, we have yet to answer one fundamental question: What can you do for your headache pain before you see your doctor or between physician visits?

This is not a simple question to answer. At times in our practice, patients call us late in the evening, early in the morning, before and after office hours because they are suffering from excruciating migraine pain. They want relief, and they want it right away. Our patients understand that if the migraine is left untreated, it can escalate and ultimately become a crisis. At times, the pain is unbearable, and the additional medical processes that accompany the migraine pain—stomach upset, fatigue, malaise, confusion, and sometimes even more serious problems such as stroke or altered level of consciousness—can be quite problematic. Many patients have already learned that a visit to the emergency room is much less than satisfactory; the bright lights, the loud noise, the scorn with which they are often greeted only make their headache pain that much worse. And visiting the doctor's office every time a migraine begins is extremely impractical. The expense—not just money, but time away from work or home and any "downtime"—required for medical office intervention can be significant. This makes it impractical to rely on your physician for migraine management, or at least for the everyday management of migraine headache pain.

This chapter is therefore designed for those who want to take an active approach to managing their migraine pain. We do not specifically endorse any one treatment modality over another, but are open to the concept of a multidisciplinary and oftentimes team approach to pain management.

Indeed, we like to use this analogy: "If you have only a hammer in your toolbox, then everything you see must look like a nail; if you have a variety of tools in your toolbox, you can take care of many different problems."

With this in mind, we dedicate this chapter to those who want to take a much more active role in their headache pain management and in treatments unrelated to prescription medications. We discuss a variety of approaches to provide a wide selection of tools that may help you combat your headache pain. You will learn about various interventions, including manual medicine, relaxation therapies, magnet therapies, and mechanical and adaptive devices; and you will even be introduced to some alternative medical systems for the treatment of migraine pain.

Because the therapeutic intervention of biofeedback is extremely important in the treatment of headache disorders, we will devote all of chapter 12 to this well-respected non-medication approach for pain management. You will learn how biofeedback relates not only to improved relaxation, but also to the treatment of headache pain. This treatment has been reviewed by the National Headache Foundation, and we feel that this certainly deserves considerable attention.

Note: We expect that our readers will not utilize any single treatment option exclusively, and will certainly not treat themselves without the supervision of a skilled physician. We espouse the concept of a multidisciplinary team approach, and that all medical care—whether traditional or alternative—be coordinated with the full understanding of your primary treating physician.

We wish to point out that, although alternative and complementary medicine has been around for thousands of years, it has only recently been approved by the American Medical Association, as well as the National Institute of Health. Indeed, almost every culture includes a concept and understanding of ritual, prayer, and reliance upon what nature provides to treat all forms of illness. The division of complementary and alternative medicine, under the supervision of the National Institute of Health, is one of the fastest growing divisions in traditional medicine today. We feel that a blending of complementary and traditional medicine is clearly the best approach to the overall treatment of our patients. We therefore dedicate this chapter to a review of these approaches, particularly to how they relate to headache pain management.

RELAXATION THERAPIES

Breathing Techniques

If you are alive, sitting or standing, and reading this book, you probably think you know how to breathe, right? The important question, however, is this: Do you know how to breathe correctly?

Breathing is something we all take for granted. Yet this seemingly simple physiologic function can often affect not only how we feel, but how we tolerate our day-to-day activities, and more importantly for migraine sufferers, how we tolerate our headache/migraine flareups.

Breathing is controlled by the autonomicor parasympathetic nervous system. It is not a function that we routinely concentrate on because our brainstem controls for us the rate of breathing, the depth of inspiration and expiration, and the overall mechanics of breathing. Unfortunately, during an acute migraine attack, one's breathing pattern is often disrupted. Frequently, the breathing pattern is accelerated with rapid, shallow respirations. This can lead to alterations in body and blood chemistries that can perpetuate this cycle of blood vessel spasm in the brain and chemical toxins circulated throughout the body, which can ultimately aggravate your headache pain syndrome. Breathing incorrectly can actually reinforce the pain syndrome, which is something no migraine sufferer wants to have happen.

However, we can actually correct our overall breathing process through a feedback mechanism to the brain and brainstem. Breathing correctly can have a positive impact on other body functions, such as heart rate, pulse, blood pressure, and stomach and intestinal function. We can slow down or reverse the nausea that often accompanies a migraine, and even reduce the pain messages that are sent to the brain. Breathing correctly can be a first line of defense in the management of acute migraine pain.

How does one breathe correctly? During a migraine attack, one of the events that occurs is a "dumping" of brain chemicals. One of these chemicals, adrenalin, is a key component in our "fight or flight" nervous system. The more adrenalin we have, the more "revved up" we are. As a result of this, we often experience a rapid heart rate, a shallow breathing pattern, and improper use of the lung muscles (diaphragm and accessory or assistant muscles). When we use our accessory muscles, we often experience muscle tightness and increased tension around the head and neck, which can lead to discomfort and at times even muscle spasm. This spasm increases the pain, which reinforces the adrenalin system, ultimately leading to a vicious downhill cycle that can in turn lead to overproduction of breakdown products and toxins that circulate in the bloodstream.

To stop this process, we must concentrate on our breathing and learn the proper breathing techniques. A deep breathing from the diaphragm (the main lung muscle) allows you to focus on the stomach muscles and move the diaphragm slowly, in a controlled fashion. We instruct our patients to try to learn this deep breathing technique in a calm, quiet environment *when they are not having a migraine headache attack.* The more comfortable patients become with the techniques listed in this chapter, the more easily they will be able to apply any of these techniques to their headache pain management when acute attack or crisis occurs.

One expert in deep-breathing techniques illustrates the appropriate breathing fashion by having individuals place one hand on their stomach. The instructor points out that while you are taking in a deep breath, you should try to push out on the stomach muscles. While breathing slowly and steadily, with a deep inhale and a slow exhale, focus on your abdominal muscles. Repeating this cycle three or four times can prove relaxing, even when you are not experiencing a headache. We explain to our patients that each individual is unique, and that finding the right rhythm and pace right for them, rather than their trying to fit into some recommended breathing pattern, is important.

Once you have mastered this simple breathing technique, perform it immediately upon the onset of headache discomfort. If you experience any prodrome (warning) or premonition that a sick headache will be coming on, begin the deep breathing process. In addition, this is a positive protocol for relaxation therapy; therefore, we recommend that our patients set aside a few minutes two or three times a day to practice this very valuable technique. Deep breathing can actually act as a positive, preventive treatment for migraine pain.

Progressive Relaxation

This is another extremely simple and easy-to-master technique. The technique deals with contracting and relaxing muscles in a steady rhythmic fashion, starting from the tip of the toes and progressing upward to involve all the small and large muscle groups of your body. This can be combined with the deep breathing just mentioned, to improve overall function and reduce headache pain.

To start, place yourself in a calm, quiet, cool, and somewhat dark environment. While either sitting comfortably or lying down comfortably, imagine your muscles in your toes and feet contracting for a series of seconds. Very, very slowly let the muscles relax. Then, proceed with the muscles in the calves, having them contract for a series of seconds, and then slowly allowing them to relax. This process is repeated, in a steady fashion, involving the muscles of the thigh, the buttocks, the abdominal region, and the chest wall. Next, contract then relax the fingertips, the hands, the forearms, and the arms. Then contract and then relax the muscles in the shoulders and the neck, and finally the muscles of the face, jaw, and the back of the head. Focus your attention on each muscle group for a series of 10 to 20 seconds for the contraction phase, and ultimately for 30 to 60 seconds for the relaxation phase. It is important to focus intensely on the muscle group that is involved, as this intense concentration can often block out some of the migraine pain messages.

While this technique rarely provides immediate relief, it often does assist those who practice it in coping with the discomfort and severity of a migraine attack. Also, relaxing the muscles of the body (especially the head and neck) can reduce the severity of a secondary headache disorder such as muscle contraction headaches.

This technique is best utilized when practiced repeatedly prior to the migraine headache; therefore, we suggest that progressive relaxation, like the deep breathing, be practiced and mastered prior to using it for a migraine therapy.

Guided Imagery

Yet another easily mastered relaxation technique, guided imagery, can be performed by virtually anyone. For maximum effectiveness, we recommend you use the images with which you are most comfortable.

For example, Dr. Kandel had a friend in medical school who would often get extremely tense and anxious prior to examinations. Indeed, Jack would often trigger his migraine headache disorder prior to an examination, and ultimately perform less than adequately because of the severe headache pain, nausea, and difficulty with concentration. He finally mastered this simple technique. Because his religious preferences did not allow Jack to fully appreciate hypnotherapy, he used guided imagery instead. He was able to visualize playing an entire baseball game as soon as he realized that a migraine was coming on. Often, by just relaxing, using deep breathing, and intensely focusing on the very vivid images he would create in his mind, his prodrome or premonition of migraine would wane, resolve, and within a matter of minutes he would not experience a headache syndrome.

Many people imagine simpler images, such as riding on a cloud, being carried by the wind, or floating along the waves of an ocean. They picture some safe, calm environment. Indeed, the more focused you are, the more detailed the vision in your mind becomes, and the more positive the response the brain can elicit. Practitioners of guided imagery who reach mastery can often control their heart rate, their breathing pattern, and even their body temperature. This all can have a positive effect on muscle contraction and prevent the negative and physiologic consequences of migraine pain.

Guided imagery, just like deep breathing and progressive relaxation, should be practiced away from the acute migraine attack during pain-free interval periods. Once mastered, this can become quite a powerful tool in the treatment of migraine headache pain.

Meditation

Meditation is yet another type of relaxation therapy. When you are able to bring your awareness to a tone, sound, phrase, or image, it is a natural consequence that your focus moves away from headache, neck pain, and migraine pain.

Meditation is extremely effective in alleviating pain, as well as reducing stress, increasing body energy, and producing an overall sense of common well-being. Positive physiologic changes that have been seen with meditation include a slower, more regulated heart rate, a more restful breathing pattern, alteration of body temperature, as well as changes in body metabolism. Some scientific studies have shown that meditation, performed correctly, can actually alter brain wave patterns. Individuals can often have a more organized brain rhythm as seen on electroencephalograms, can have a deeper state of relaxation, and more focused attention. In addition, individuals who are skilled at meditation often have improved and prolonged attention, and have performed better in testing situations. In addition, chemical studies have found that meditation often produces a higher circulating level of the body's relaxation chemicals.

Research studies have also found a number of positive effects of meditation. These include improved energy, vigor, decreased fatigue, increased stamina, and an improvement in a patient's self-rating of headache pain. Individuals who meditate frequently often describe their sleep cycle as more restful, more natural, with more rapid onset of restful sleep. In addition, those who meditate on a frequent basis often claim to reduce their negative habits, such as use of alcohol, caffeine, and tobacco. For purposes of migraine pain management, however, the most important aspect of meditation is that studies have revealed that meditation is effective in reducing pain.

There are several meditation techniques. Most instructors initially attempt to train individuals in a group setting. This is important, as you will want the support, the reassurance, and the encouragement of others as you begin to meditate. The meditation process requires anywhere from just a few minutes to as long as 30- to 40-minute sessions, depending on your skill and your desired level of effects. Meditation does require training, and we recommend you work with a meditation specialist who can help you learn appropriate techniques, as well as help you monitor your body functions to determine whether you are achieving the proper goals.

In essence, the meditator makes a focused effort to concentrate on one single imaged thought or idea—possibly one physical function, such as your breathing, a specific noise or sound, or a particular body stimulus. You have probably heard of people reciting a mantra, which is a recited formula designed to produce a particular effect. Meditators use this technique to move their attention away from the external world by focusing on this phrase or word by repeating it.

In essence, the concept is to quiet the mind, allowing it to filter out the body's distractions. If you stop and think for just one moment of all the information the body has to take in, you'll realize your body has to receive, adapt to, and filter thousands of sensory inputs on a moment-to-moment basis. Although initially believed to have risen in Eastern religious practices, meditation exists in essentially all cultures. Certainly Christian practices such as repeating "Hail Mary's" may be identified as one form of meditation. In addition, various physical activities—such as concentration in sports, as well as various exercise techniques—can be viewed as reaching that sense of focused attention required for changing physiologic function of the body.

One form, transcendental meditation, has been studied by various professionals who have found that it leads to a number of positive responses such as reduced health-care usage, increased longevity, increased individual rating for quality of life, and reduction of pain.

Individuals who practice transcendental meditation also appear to have less anxiety and stress; decreased incidence of such pathologic processes as high cholesterol, high blood pressure, substance use; and increased attention.

As with everything, old concepts and techniques have been modified over the years. A current popular buzzword, "stress management," means nothing more than reducing external stressors in order to reduce the negative impact on body function and to achieve improved health.

Yoga

If the word "yoga" brings to mind images of an individual wearing a loincloth and contorting his or her body into impossible positions, you might want to rethink this concept. Achieving a state of acrobatic agility is not the primary function or goal of yoga therapy. Indeed, yoga comes from the Sanskrit work "yuj" which means to fix together or harness the mind, body, and breathing of an individual into perfect balance. Yoga applies to the achievement of balance in three different arenas. The first is the physical, which is what brings to mind the various postures (called "asanas"). The various postures have been determined to actually help to relax and tone the muscles, as well to provide deep massage to the inner muscles. The second aspect of yoga is the breathing exercises (called "pranayama"). These are the slow, appropriate breathing techniques that restore the body's vital energies. The third aspect of yoga is the role of meditation, which aims to quiet the mind from all of life's busyness, as listed previously.

There are many types of yoga, and a variety of forms, but the two most popular are "Raja Yoga" and "Hatha Yoga." Raja refers to the yoga therapy that focuses on the mind. This is consistent with the prior relaxation therapies that we have already discussed.

Hatha is the yoga of willpower, and this attempts to help reach a spiritual cleansing through refocusing the body's energy centers. As mentioned, yoga can take many techniques, and is certainly most appropriately used for migraine prevention when it is fully mastered. It would be difficult to initiate yoga therapy for the first time in the throes of the sick, nauseating migraine. However, if one has become adept at performing these therapies—stretching, breathing, and meditation processes—singly or in a combined fashion, they can be quite powerful tools to refocus the body's attention from the migraine onto more positive images.

Tai Chi

Tai Chi is actually an abbreviation of "Tai Chi Ch'uan," a Chinese martial art therapy. It is quite effective at bringing balance back to the body, both in a physical and spiritual sense. Tai Chi is performed by following a series of very disciplined and discrete movements that unite the mind and body, and which have been found to provide a number of positive physiologic benefits as well.

Although this form of relaxation therapy is best known as a variation on martial arts and self-defense therapy, it is much more than just a form of fighting. Tai Chi is also a form of internal therapy, which focuses on control, relaxation, and is a highly focused form of meditation. Indeed, some have coined the term "fluid meditation" in reference to Tai Chi as meditation associated with motion or movement.

Scientific studies have found that Tai Chi is extremely effective in improving a multitude of physical processes, including Parkinson's disease, balance difficulties, arthritis, back problems, and blood pressure abnormalities. In addition, Tai Chi is very effective in reducing pain, as well as in relaxing muscle tension. Because tension is a key characteristic of migraine syndrome, Tai Chi can be extremely effective in reducing the muscle contraction component of migraine headache disorders.

While this technique does take time, training, and a great deal of effort to learn, the benefits can certainly be worth it. A number of books through which you can learn the discrete Tai Chi movements are available at most local libraries. Tai Chi has "made it into the mainstream" because it is of particular benefit to individuals who have a difficult time with aerobic activity and exercise in general, but who want to gain the benefits of an exercise program.

Once mastered, Tai Chi is an extremely valuable form of relaxation therapy.

Hypnosis

Unfortunately, this relaxation therapy has been sorely misrepresented by the Hollywood movie culture. When first approached with the concept of hypnosis, most patients fear they are being put "under someone's spell" and will be forced to perform acts they would normally never do. This could not be further from the truth. In truth, all hypnosis is "self-hypnosis," a wonderful technique that allows you to take control of your own mind and achieve a state of focused attention.

As mentioned, hypnosis is always performed and controlled by the patient. The therapist acts only as a guide, and often as an instructor to initially educate individuals on how to perform hypnosis. It is impossible to be hypnotized "against your will."

Hypnosis therapy, which dates back to the ancient Greeks, originates from the word "hypnos," meaning sleep. Inductions into tranced states with the appropriate positive therapeutic benefits were a central feature of early Greek healing, and subsequent variations on hypnotic trances have been used throughout the centuries. Hypnosis in the modern form began in the eighteenth century when Franz Mesmer used "magnetic healing" (his term for hypnosis) to treat a variety of medical disorders. The famed Austrian neurologist Sigmund Freud also used hypnosis. Unfortunately, as a variety of emotions emerged under the treatment, he abandoned hypnosis for his more traditional "Freudian therapy." Hypnosis was popular prior to the introduction of anesthesia, and was in fact a preferred method of pain management, with many minor and some major surgeries performed under hypnosis. Today, hypnosis is more often used for addiction therapy, for cessation of habits such as smoking and drug use, as well as for behavior control. Treatment of anxiety or phobias in the control of pain (including migraine) has been the focus of current hypnosis treatment.

What is hypnosis? Like other forms of relaxation therapy, hypnosis is a form of focused and highly directed concentration. In this state of concentration, individuals are indeed highly suggestible. Physiologically, hypnosis resembles very deep relaxation, as measured by changes in the autonomic or sympathetic nervous system, changes in oxygen flow, changes in galvanic skin response (the measurement of electrical conductivity in the surface of the skin), and more organized brain wave activity. Many physicians of various backgrounds are actively involved in The American Society for Clinical Hypnosis.

With regard to pain management, twelve controlled studies, reviewed by the National Institute of Health, have demonstrated hypnosis as a superior way to reduce headache pain syndrome in children and teenagers.

Children in one study were given either placebo (sugar pill), propranolol (a blood pressure medicine used to prevent migraine), or self-hypnosis. The children who were taught self-hypnosis experienced a reduction in the severity and frequency of headaches. Another group experienced dramatic improvement in subjective rating of pain, with those trained in hypnotherapy able to tolerate their headache pain much more easily than those who do not receive hypnosis intervention.

Hypnotherapy is often used as a reserve or "second line" therapy when conventional medication and medicine treatments fail. However, it is clear from research as well as patient response that hypnotherapy may be an ideal first-line treatment for controlling and ultimately preventing migraine pain syndromes, as well as a variety of additional headache pains.

Like other forms of relaxation therapy, hypnosis can take some time to master. We urge our patients to *be* patient and to practice until hypnosis becomes easier with each session. Ultimately, individuals should be able to enter into a mild tranced state in a very short period of time, within seconds to one minute. Periodic practice of this treatment modality can lead to very positive long-term clinical results, not only in migraine pain management, but also in a general sense of wellness and well-being.

MANUAL THERAPIES

In this section, we will review a number of manual hands-on approaches, which over the centuries have been practiced by various cultures to provide pain relief. An important element in all these forms of manual healing is the art of touching—the need for patients to touch others and to be touched. Under the category of manual therapies we include treatment forms of massage, manipulation therapy, pressure point therapy, acupuncture, and acupressure. All are a variation on the art of healing using a manual approach; any one form of treatments could (and often does) encompass an entire text.

Therapeutic Massage

Hippocrates, the master physician who is considered the Father of Medicine, is noted for this statement: "The physician must be experienced in many things, but most assuredly in rubbing." The need to be touched or rubbed where one hurts is basic. It is an instinct, just like eating and sleeping, to fulfill primitive body needs. Remote cave paintings from over 15,000 years ago reveal individuals being treated with massage. A Chinese medical text over 4,000 years old outlined therapeutic treatment with massage. Massage therapy has been espoused as an appropriate treatment by a number of historic physicians, including Salsas, Galen, and a number of more noted modern physicians (Kandel and Sudderth: *Back Pain, What Works*, and *The Arthritis Solution*).

Massage therapy has made a resurgence as an appropriate treatment protocol over the last decade or two. Now all 50 states offer certification examinations, and over 80 different approaches and methods have been classified as massage therapy over the last 20 years.

The more recognized massage therapy treatment, "Swedish massage," uses a system of long strokes, kneading, mild friction, and pressure therapy. The therapy is usually applied in the direction of blood flow toward the heart, with the masseuse often massaging muscles associated with active and passive movements at the joints. The Swedish massage is frequently focused on general relaxation, which is helpful in relieving tension and reducing stress.

Deep tissue massage is more focused on chronic pain management—reducing muscle tension—as is evident by the treatment of direct pressure release, slow strokes, and friction across muscle planes. It is usually performed with a much greater pressure as compared to the lighter Swedish massage.

Neuromuscular massage is a newer type of therapy intended to increase blood flow and reduce muscle cramping and muscle spasm. It is often effective in releasing trigger points, and in releasing pressure, tension, and entrapment of nerves caused by soft tissue contraction. Pressure point massage and myofascial release are often variations of neuro-muscular massage.

But how does massage work? It appears to have a three-pronged mechanism of action, any one of which can be beneficial in reducing headache pain. We feel that it is the combination of all three actions that brings out the most positive outcome.

First, therapeutic massage is inherently relaxing for patients. By simply presenting themselves for massage, myofascial release, and manipulative care, our patients are removing themselves from the routine environment, placing themselves under a non-stressful, darkened, quiet, calm, and relaxing environment. This change alone has positive effects. It can remove possible headache triggers, remove exogenous and environmental stressors, and allow patients to refocus on pain reduction rather than on their daily life stressors and their routine environment.

Second, the preparation for therapeutic massage and the act of actually receiving massage is usually relaxing. It can reduce stress and anxiety. Anyone who has suffered a severe migraine headache can testify that the acute anxiety associated with the headache itself is a major problem when a migraine symptom first presents. Anxiety escalating questions—"Oh no! Am I going to get sick? Will I have to leave work? Will I have to stop what I am doing?"—are inevitable for many migraine sufferers. This anxiety can then lead to a rebound phenomenon, with additional release of stress chemicals (catecholamines, adrenalin) and a buildup of toxins and waste products. These often result from prolonged muscle contraction, muscle spasm, tissue breakdown, and release of lactic acid and other such toxins into the system.

All these factors taken together further aggravate the headache pain. By reducing the anxiety, on the other hand, one can also reduce the adrenalin and stress chemicals that are often associated with anxiety. This in turn often leads to a reduction in pain and certainly can also reduce the severity and duration of the headache.

The third, and possibly the most effective mechanism of action and therapeutic massage, is the physical trigger release, myofascial release, and the direct muscle anti-inflammatory effect of the massage itself.

The actual massage can break down tissue triggers that are also frequently seen in both migraine and chronic daily headache sufferers. In addition, we often see improved flexibility and range of motion, decreased spasm and muscle triggers (mini-spasm in the muscle) in direct response to therapeutic massage.

A focal massage over the neck and shoulder region can help reduce local triggers. This procedure can enable the other body muscles to relax. As a result, muscle tightening throughout the body is avoided. Massage as a healing therapy works by improving circulation in and around the muscles. This eliminates the buildup of waste products and toxins such as lactic acid. With the removal or avoidance of these waste products, the muscles that are overworked, tense, and contracted can relax; and ultimately one can break the headache cycle.

We point out that just as every physician is different, every massage therapist is different. If there are individual techniques, practices, or protocols that seem to work better for you, communicating this to your therapist is essential.

You should also avoid techniques that seem to increase pain or discomfort, and again should communicate this information to the massage therapist. Remember, therapeutic intervention is a team approach, and you need to be an active member of the team.

CHIROPRACTIC CARE

Chiropractic care, a unique practice of medicine, has recently celebrated its centennial, which means over 100 years of effective and appropriate therapeutic intervention by chiropractic physicians. This is the science concerned with the relationship between structure, particularly of the spine, and function, predominantly of the central and peripheral nervous system. The concept of balance as it relates to the spinal column and nervous system is addressed through chiropractic manipulation, adjustments, and intervention. The chiropractic philosophy involves these four major tenets:

1. The human body has a unique and innate ability to re-focus and balance itself, and given half the chance, the body can heal almost anything.
2. The nervous system is extremely highly developed in humans, and influences all other body systems.
3. The presence of joint dysfunction, as well as subluxation or changes in the spinal column anatomy may interfere with the neuromuscular skeletal system, and may ultimately have a negative impact on neurologic function and body function.
4. Chiropractic physicians' ability to treat is based on the ability to diagnosis improper structural changes, dysfunction and to realign the spinal column to allow for physiologic healing.

The chiropractic profession was founded in the 1890s, when David Palmer, the magnetic healer, applied his knowledge to treating patients, particularly a local janitor. Palmer was the first one to actually use the spinal column and its projections as levers to adjust the spinal column. Palmer is known as the founder of chiropractic care, and addresses the treatment modalities of subluxation and joint manipulation for symptom relief. Chiropractic care has gone through an evolution, to now include not only subluxation and adjustment therapy as treatment for all disease processes, but also to include a more encompassing approach of health and wellness. This includes a broad-based educational program, involving basic and clinical sciences, laboratory work, dissection, and clinical care. There are a variety of chiropractic techniques, all under the "umbrella of chiropractic care." These include the following: sacral occipital technique, activator technique, diversified technique, terminal point technique, flexion distraction therapy, Gonstead technique, and applied kinesiology, as well as the multidisciplinary approach combining the above-listed techniques, which most modern-day chiropractic physicians use.

Chiropractors generally follow a set of guidelines, "The Mercy Conference Guidelines," that are meant to be an overall guide to chiropractic care rather than a definitive protocol for chiropractic treatment. Chiropractic care has been one of the largest and fastest-growing segments of the complementary and alternative medical division, with chiropractic physicians seeing approximately 15% of the U.S. population, almost all in private office settings. The chiropractic education program is routinely a five-year curriculum, and incorporates a multitude of intervention, including anatomy, pathology, manual techniques, chemistry, and physics, all of which are under the supervision of the Council of Chiropractic Education.

With regard to low back pain, studies show that patients relate chiropractic care as more effective, and in many instances more cost-effective, than orthopedic intervention, physical therapy intervention, or neurosurgical intervention.

In our practice, we have found that a combined therapy approach between medication management of our patients and chiropractic care has been extremely effective, particularly for patients who suffer from both migraine headache disorder and muscle contraction or tension-type headaches. We have found chiropractic care to be an extremely safe and effective treatment for soft tissue pain, myofascial pain, and a variety of joint pain syndromes.

Without medication usage, and with proper spinal adjustment performed in the hands of a competent and certified chiropractic physician, the treatment can be a very positive experience that produces outstanding pain relief for the patient. It is important to note that chiropractic physicians with whom we work are also highly educated on wellness and health education. These physicians also provide additional information about the patient's activity, which may actually improve overall wellness and reduce destructive behaviors that can act as migraine triggers.

While there have been anecdotal reports of major mishaps with chiropractic care, these are indeed anecdotal. Careful review of the literature has revealed chiropractic care to be extremely safe, indeed safer than a trip to the local beauty parlor when it comes to stroke or a serious pathologic outcome. We encourage our patients to be informed, and find that patients who are reluctant to proceed with chiropractic care are those who lack a clear understanding of the practice and potential benefits of chiropractic treatment.

Pressure Point Therapies

This concept of therapeutic intervention is based on Eastern medicine. It is the concept of using finger pressure on specific points, usually affiliated with various meridians (points of energy flow, mapped out in a variety of Oriental medicine practices). In addition, trigger point therapies are focused on releasing neurologic triggers to reduce pain; improve function, range of motion, flexibility; and reduce various disease states. Massage therapy, as mentioned earlier in the chapter, is a natural offshoot from earlier pressure point therapy.

One popular therapy is reflexology, which is based on the concept that specific zones on the feet are related to various body organs, body systems. This is a concept of zone therapy, where pressure release on various aspects of the feet releases a variety of painful syndromes. Treatment of headache pain, neck pain, stroke, sinusitis, and sciatica, as well as menstrual cramping, are all seen with this type of therapy.

There are a variety of Chinese trigger point therapies, which include energizing and relaxing techniques. Variations of these therapies include "Ma" (the rubbing of various body rubs with the palmar fingertips), "Pi" (tapping with the palmar fingertips), "Tao" (pinching with the thumb and the fingertip),

"An" (rhythmical pressing with the thumb, palm, or the entire clenched hand), "Ning" (pinching and lifting motion), and "Tui" (pushing, often associated with vibration type approach). These techniques are used in combination to relieve muscle pressures, and can be addressed for a variety of symptoms; but for our purposes, we focus on the use of these modalities for treatment of headache, migraine, stiff neck, and pain.

Yet another form of pressure point therapy includes acupressure treatments. This also relates to following meridian points, or accupoints, with either stimulation or relaxation approach. It is beyond the scope of this chapter to outline the various types of acupressure treatment; it is clear that there are a wide variety of these approaches. Indeed, a generalized concept is that energy focuses in the feet, hands, or ears, with many acupuncture and acupressure points located in these regions. The belief is that these therapeutic interventions release various neurotransmitters, which travel along the nerve lines or meridians, and ultimately affect a variety of processes. Treatment, and release of these pressure points, can ultimately result in improved health, beyond just the pain relief.

Acupuncture

Some doctors refuse to believe that nontraditional therapeutic interventions can play a positive role in pain relief; we, on the other hand, have seen therapeutic benefits with acupuncture intervention.

Acupuncture, an ancient Eastern treatment, can lead to release of the body's own pain "relievers," endorphins and cephalins. These chemicals are our own personal morphine and opiate-like substances, released by the body when we experience pain. In addition, they are released by long-distance runners during a race, allowing them to experience the euphoria of the marathon run.

Researchers don't fully understand how acupuncture works. However, scientific studies have revealed that when patients were given a chemical agent that blocks morphine (such as naloxone or natrexone), the chemical also appeared to completely block the effects of acupuncture therapy. This means that the body's own pain chemicals were either not released or the chemical receptors they are trying to act upon are saturated with the blocking medicines.

Eastern medical practitioners have used acupuncture for many years, to provide pain relief and pain blocking. In some cases, acupuncture has even been used to block pain during surgical procedures.

Acupuncture may also affect the gastrointestinal (stomach and intestine) system. As discussed earlier, the bowel and stomach functions slow during the onset of an acute migraine; the stomach may become nearly paralyzed. Acupuncture seems to overcome this "gastroparesis," thus leading to a significant reduction of the nausea of the migraine headache.

MAGNETIC THERAPY

Everything old seems new again. This applies to attitudes, fashion, diets, and just about everything in which we take part. The use of magnets for therapeutic purposes is no exception. Cleopatra wore magnetic bracelets, anklets, or amulets thousands of years ago. She is only one of many who believed in the power of magnetic therapy to reduce pain and speed the healing process. Today, some people are convinced that they have "discovered" the therapeutic benefit of magnetic treatment.

Magnetic therapy uses the concept of biologically active and effective magnets. This is not the simple north-south directed polarity. It is a different type of magnetic field. According to the concept of biologically active magnets, it is predominately negative polarity that seems to improve healing. This is true not only for the individual cellular level, but also for the total body.

Most of us have had a positive "magnetic experience." For example, the last time you sat by a quiet stream or brook, or in front of the ocean's pounding surf, you most likely felt calm, relaxed, and refreshed as the day's cares floated away. Why? Is it just the water, or is there something else? One theory holds that increased positive and negative ions surround these bubbling brooks and flowing streams, and in some way these enhance our own body's energy fields. They are thought to provide positive energy, restore our sense of wellness, and rebalance our body.

Similarly, when we sit in an oxygen-enriched environment, such as a forest, we also seem to be refreshed. Some theorize that the increased oxygen content of the air, along with the increase in positive magnetic ions, provides for the greatest supply of oxygen-enriched blood cells coursing through our body. This allows more nutrition, more oxygen, and more energy to each individual cell and to the muscles and joints in general. Apparently, this can lead to decreased pain and increased mobility. This can also lead to an increased sense of wellness, and be quite effective in preventing headache syndrome, migraine syndrome, and overall muscle-contraction headaches.

Is there any scientific evidence that magnetic therapy can actually work? At the Johns Hopkins Treatment Pain Center, researchers performed a controlled study on magnetic therapy. In this study, some patients with chronic pain received placebo therapy (like a sugar pill), while other individuals were provided magnetic therapy. Initially, both groups of patients improved. The individuals using placebo therapy improved slightly, but this effect rapidly tapered off. Those who received the magnets, however, showed dramatic improvement. They had increased function, increased range of motion, decreased pain, and their subjective rating of their pain remained reduced. The fact that those who receive magnetic therapy have no negative side effects makes this a very reasonable choice for individuals who have either failed traditional therapy or have rejected it.

It should be pointed out, however, that some types of magnetic treatment may not be free of side effects. For example, right now there is medical controversy as to whether or not high pulsating magnetic pollution, such as that seen around high-powered transmission lines, can produce harmful side effects. While this has not been proven, a number of anecdotal studies and case reports have been cited, mentioning such problems as memory loss, headaches, changes in heart rhythm, and altered blood chemistry. This will require further study in the future.

Uses of Magnetic Therapy

How do physicians use magnetic therapy? One orthopedic surgeon has used magnetic therapy in combination with traditional surgical intervention. Healing for bone fracture, particularly poorly connected bones, has been discovered to be greater than 80%, while traditional rates (40–50% without the use of magnetic therapy) are much lower. Magnetic science has made a huge impact in traditional medicine. All physicians value the benefits of magnetic science, particularly as utilized through magnetic resonant imaging (MRI) scanners. Orthopedic surgeons have found that this improved bone healing in their difficult-to-treat fracture patients. Of interest, the University of Miami, Florida, Department of Orthopedics is now routinely using magnet therapy for patients with fractures (Dr. Kandel, personal communication). These machines provide powerful diagnostic information daily on a variety of illnesses. MRIs are very important for assessing brain function, neck function, spinal cord involvement, and disc disease of the neck. They are also important in ruling out such significant conditions as disorders of the nervous system, tumors, and pressure on the brain. It is interesting that many traditional physicians are skeptical when the topic comes up of adjusting this magnetic polarity for therapeutic intervention rather than for diagnostic testing.

As this is a "new field" of medical science, there is little more than multiple anecdotal stories at this time. We hear, for example, of athletes who have increased their stamina, exercise, and even their weight-lifting or weight-training ability, using the benefits of magnetic therapy. A recent article in *American Pain Journal* describes how magnetic therapy may be helpful for a variety of neurologic illnesses such as neuropathy, which is the inflammation of the small nerve twigs often found in the lower extremities.

Anecdotal Stories

As traditional physicians, we understand that anecdotal stories are not the same as proven scientific research. However, we do not deny the value of information, received from even a single patient, in terms of providing insight into the potential benefits of this mode of therapy. John, a patient of Dr. Kandel, had been bedridden for three days with severe intractable migraine headache pain. Because he was unable to tolerate traditional medications due to medicine intolerance, gastrointestinal symptoms, and prior ulcer disease, John had sought treatment using alternative intervention. He had tried a variety of treatments, including manual therapies, as well as heat and ice and various relaxation techniques. Nothing seemed to work. However, a friend who heard of John's plight provided local magnetic pads, which John placed over the base of his skull, and a magnetic mattress. John also received two magnetic rollers to be used over the neck muscles, the base of the skull, and the shoulder region.

A delighted John contacted the office, stating that he had found a "cure" for his headache pain without medications. Apparently, by using the magnetic mattress and the pads and rollers, he had improved his neck and head pain syndrome. His nausea had improved, the range of motion of his neck improved, and indeed, to this day he has used the magnetic treatment for recurrence of his migraine disorder. While he has not gained complete control of his headache syndrome, certainly the frequency of headaches, as well as severity of his headache syndrome, has remarkably reduced.

Another theory of magnetic treatment involves utilizing the magnetic pads over meridians or acupuncture points. In this way, magnetic therapy may be a variant of magnetic acupressure. This seems to be very effective for reducing muscle tension and muscle contraction in the larger muscles and ligaments, as well as reducing joint pain.

Neurologists in general have been treating individuals with facial pain, cranial facial pain, and head pain for many years. This type of disorder is often very difficult to treat. We've discovered in our practice that a variety of treatments—including medications, antidepressant medicines, and electrostimulation—along with a combination of magnetic therapy, lead to significant improvement.

Magnets have been studied for their effects on various areas of the body, including headache pain and neck pain. Apparently, individual results seem to vary significantly, based on location, size of area, and patient's attitude. Patients with a positive attitude seem to correlate with an improved response rate, while those who doubt the benefits of magnetic therapy respond less well. We've discovered in our practice that magnetic therapy seems to provide many individuals an effective treatment or modality, with minimal or no negative side effects.

Types of Magnets

Magnets marketed by many different companies now come in several strengths and sizes. We have had our greatest success with Nikken magnetic pads. These come in small strips, can be localized over trigger points, and larger strips can be placed over the neck muscles and over the shoulder girdle. (Note: We are not distributors, nor do we have any financial interest in this or any magnetic products.)

We have found magnetic balls to be useful for relaxation techniques and for hand therapy, very much like traditional hand therapy for arthritis joint pain. Adding the magnetic strips to the base of the skull and along the muscles of the neck seems to improve range of motion, increase flexibility, reduce pain, and reduce the frequency and severity of headaches. This seems to lead to an overall subjective improvement in pain, a subjective rating of increased warmth, and more rapid onset of pain relief. Overall, the frequency of headache episodes and the severity or intensity of the headache event seems to be reduced with the use of magnetic therapy.

Is magnetic therapy expensive? As health-care expenses go, magnetic therapy can run the gamut from relatively inexpensive to moderately expensive. However, favorite forms of magnetic treatment are "mag steps," a relatively low-cost item. For just over $60, these large oversized shoe inserts, with bumps on one side and indentations on the other, can be effective in improving a general sense of wellness. As we discussed earlier, with the concept of reflexology (local stimulation of the feet), these seem to improve overall health. This may be the mechanism of action for mag steps.

At the other end of the spectrum are magnetic bed pads, which range in cost from $450 to more than $600. When multiple body areas are involved, such as in our patients with fibromyalgia, this may be a reasonable option. However, we suggest that our patients start small, with the magnetic rollers, magnetic strips, or magnetic footpads. Based on individual results, we then recommend additional intervention, as appropriate.

The Bottom Line

This said, we must admit we still don't fully understand the mechanism of magnet therapy, how it works, or even why it works. We simply see the results in a number of our patients.

Those who practice only traditional medicine tend to belittle magnetic therapy as sham or placebo treatment. When we hear this, we smile and point out that the proof is in the patient care and patient results. Some who have failed a number of traditional treatments try magnetic therapy and do well, feel better, and point to their success. We feel that we are actually treating a person's illness, rather than an illness in a person.

Possibly, we appreciate magnetic therapy because it makes patients actively involved participants in their own health care. Because the physician cannot always be there when a migraine has its onset, the patient who is an ally, rather than passive observer of his or her health care, is much more likely to find relief.

In addition, the patients who are willing to go through a routine, bother to put on magnetic pads, place the magnetic rollers in place, and apply the proper techniques are often reminded to use proper body mechanics, be aware of proper breathing techniques, and follow through with additional physician instructions. These can be as simple as stretching and flexibility, deep breathing, or relaxation techniques. This multidisciplinary approach to pain—magnetic therapy used in conjunction with additional treatment modalities—is in itself a benefit perhaps worth the cost of magnetic therapy.

MECHANICAL DEVICES AND OTHER ADAPTIVE INTERVENTIONS

Headband Therapy

A special headache headband, designed and marketed by California physician Dr. Vijayn, has provided relief to some migraineurs. Where local pressure and ice packs have failed, Dr. Vijayn found that applying pressure to the area of pain with an elastic headband secured with Velcro or rubber provided excellent headache relief.

The headband method can be used along with pain medication and vasoconstrictor agents (medicines that cause the blood vessels to narrow), although neither is required.

Although it is not clear how pain relief was obtained, the headband was found to work for patients, according to a report in the medical journal *Headache*. Most patients, however, needed to keep the headband in place throughout the course of the headache; if they took it off, the headache came back.

This treatment seems both safe and effective, with limited or no potential side effects. Some of our patients have combined this therapeutic modality with the use of magnets, placing the magnetic discs or pads beneath the headband. Again, our patients have reported even greater relief when using the two treatments in combination.

Transcutaneous Electrical Nerve Stimulation (TENS Therapy)

The TENS unit is a small battery-operated device that provides electric stimulation to the affected limbs and joints of headache sufferers. (Transcutaneous means "passing through the skin.")

There are various ideas and rationales regarding how this treatment works. Some involve release of endorphins, activating acupuncture meridian pathways, or possibly overstimulation of nerve endings. In our earlier discussion on pain, we discussed the fact that all pain messages must be related to the brain. If the stimulator produces an intense sensation of numbness and pressure, this numbness message may arrive at the brain first, and effectively block the pain messages carried in on small fibers. This is actually the "gating theory" of pain management.

While TENS therapy may not be effective for acute headache pain, it has been proven to be a safe, relatively effective therapy for the muscle contraction component of headache disorders. In addition, patients who have jaw joint discomfort (TMJ), which acts as one trigger for headache disorders, can be effectively treated with these TENS pads placed directly over the muscles surrounding the jaw joints.

If there is any electric rhythm disturbance in your body, or if you have a cardiac pacemaker, be sure to first discuss electrical stimulation therapy with your physician. In addition, because the literature regarding the use of electric stimulation on pregnant women is mixed, pregnant women should ask their doctors whether this therapy is appropriate. The TENS unit comes as a battery pack, which looks very much like a pager with attached electrodes. These electrodes are attached to pads, which are applied to the muscles and joints around the head and neck. If you live in a hot climate or tend to sweat easily or have oily skin, the pads may not stick well, and you may not get the desired therapeutic result.

A new version of the electric stimulator is the Sol TENS, a hand-held electric stimulator device. Our patients seem to like this device more than the traditional unit, as they can be more active participants in their pain management. The Sol TENS is a probe that allows users to pick up muscle and joint triggers in and around the head and neck. It can be used over the temple muscles, over the jaw, or over the base of the skull. The unit is accompanied by a booklet providing acupressure and meridian information to increase its effectiveness. Many patients feel comfortable using this small device (which easily fits in a pocket or purse) rather than medications, which may have side effects.

Many of our initially skeptical physician colleagues have seen that the Sol TENS probe does indeed find the muscle trigger.

After three or four stimulation episodes, the probe will no longer find these active triggers—because they will be gone. Many patients claim significant relief from using this device, and research by the Food and Drug Administration back up such claims. It has been determined that this TENS device works for myofascial and musculoskeletal pains. This is just one more example of new medical and biotechnology treatments that will become more user-friendly, effective, and appropriate for the treatment of acute migraine and headache pain syndromes.

Home Electrical Stimulation Therapy

Electrical stimulation is very helpful for alleviating pain associated with headache disorders, which is often the result of joint and soft tissue processes, particularly inflammation and swelling. The treatment increases circulation and the patient's range of motion, particularly around the head and neck, and works by directly decreasing the pain messages as well as the inflammation. The stimulating probes send out electric information, which then sends pulses to nerve endings. This process blocks the flow of pain messages to the nervous system, thereby producing analgesia or pain relief. In addition, the electric probe can actually stimulate the release of endorphins (the brain's painkiller chemicals), which again decreases pain.

Electrical stimulation is similar to TENS therapy, which was discussed above. However, it is performed using more potent (and unfortunately expensive) equipment, and has routinely been used under a physical therapist's supervision.

A variation on electrical stimulation can lead to what is known as muscle re-education. This is particularly effective for the mixed headache disorder or tension-type headache pain. Electrical stimulation through electrodes placed on muscle can actually strengthen the muscle, increase muscle tone, and allow the muscle to contract in a more appropriate fashion than previously obtained. In this manner, the muscle is being "re-educated." This technique is often used in combination with relaxation, guided imagery, or biofeedback (discussed in the next chapter). The goal is to improve muscle and joint function and ultimately to alleviate head and neck pain.

Recently, the FDA approved release of home electrical stimulation units, which are the same units most physical therapy centers use. Although a number of reputable companies provide such units, we have been particularly impressed with those provided by the Home Therapy Products Company (PGS-3000) as well as the Rx Medical Therapy Products Company, which provides another quality home electric stimulation device. One benefit of the Rx Medical home electric stimulation unit is that it has an internal counter, which can be quite helpful in monitoring the patient's compliance. With the majority of our patients, this is not an issue; however, when treatment fails, the internal monitor on the Rx Medical unit allows us to determine whether or not the patient is taking full advantage of the electric stimulation therapy, as originally intended.

The home electric stimulation units do require a prescription, but are covered by most insurance companies. We often will combine home electric stimulation therapy with other treatments. For example, we may recommend that prior to electric stimulation therapy, our patients use heat for 12 to 20 minutes, then use the electric stimulation therapy for 30 to 40 minutes, and then ultimately use a cool-down or ice program. This simulates a true physical therapy session, which can cost up to $150 at some therapy centers.

We are impressed with the progress in technology, which allows our patients to have a great deal of control with newer treatment options.

Home Cervical Traction

Another mechanical and adaptive device that is effective for some of our patients, not only for migraine but also for muscle contraction and tension-type headaches, is home cervical traction. Of the variety of traction devices available, we have found two to be more effective. One is a simple, low-cost traction unit, which uses a water bottle filled to certain levels for the appropriate weight, and hangs from the door. There is a chinstrap, which can elevate the head and neck, which performs gentle traction. By releasing the tension from the joints of the neck, by the muscles, patients can actually have some moderate to significant pain relief. This may not be appropriate for acute migraine attacks, but some of our patients have reported that using it helps them abort a migraine when the aura or premonition of a headache starts. In addition to the over-the-door water-bottle traction device, which is relatively inexpensive (approximately $30), there is a much more elaborate pneumatic device, again provided by Home Therapy Products. This includes a pneumatic pump with a soft collar, which allows the patients to lie on their back on a firm surface. This simulates a traction device used in the office, and can provide extremely controlled traction therapy for our patients. However, this device is quite a bit less portable than the water-bottle unit, and it costs quite a bit more (over $2,000). For patients who are interested in this device, we often recommend they lease or rent one for a trial period of two to three months to avoid being "stuck" with a very expensive unit that may provide minimal pain relief.

The mechanism of action for all traction therapy is the same, whether the therapy is performed by a chiropractor or osteopathic physician, or by mechanical devices. Distracting or separating the joint places less pressure on the joints, and therefore translates to less stimulation of the nerve endings. In addition, stretching the muscles, which are often quite contracted in migraine and tension headaches, can alleviate the breakdown products, toxins, and lactic acid buildup in the muscle groups. By reducing these toxins, you will experience less negative feedback, and your muscles can ultimately stay relaxed.

We find traction therapy helpful, but additional therapeutic modalities are often required to provide optimum pain relief.

CRYOTHERAPY

Cryotherapy is attracting many patient advocates. This high-tech-sounding term simply refers to the application of cold to painful areas. When you apply an ice pack, you are using cryotherapy. Patients often ask us when to use heat and when to use ice. The answer is that it depends on the injury, complaints, and the time at which these injuries or complaints occur. The use of cold or heat must be tailored to each individual's situation.

Applying cryotherapy for acute headache pain with intense inflammation is very effective. The cold closes blood vessels and leads to reduction in the chemical products (cytocrines) that start the whole inflammatory process. Penetrating cold ultimately reduces swelling. As swelling is reduced, muscle spasm is also reduced. Another advantage of using cryotherapy is that cold can act as a deep stimulation, which ultimately blocks the pathways of the small pain fibers. This theory was originated by Melzak and Wall and was a cornerstone theory in pain management.

In addition to applying ice packs to the painful joint, you can perform ice massage, which involves gently moving the ice over your skin. There is also a technique called "spray and stretch" in which ethyl chloride spray (a cooling/freezing surface anesthetic) is used on the muscles. When the muscles are numb, the muscles, ligaments, and tendons are stretched. As the muscles warm up, the cool, numb sensation usually gives rise to a burning, warm sensation of the muscle and joint. This could be repeated periodically to increase mobilization and increase the range of motion of the inflating joints.

Cryotherapy must be used in moderation. It is dangerous to leave ice on inflamed areas for more than 20 minutes. Making that mistake can result in a reactive and negative secondary process: The blood vessels involuntarily open and the ice could cause blood vessel damage. If you perform cryotherapy on a regular basis, apply the ice pack for 20 minutes, then take it off for an hour and repeat this process to the affected muscles.

While in the throes of acute migraine headache pain, placing an ice pack over the base of the skull and the top of your neck can be extremely effective in alleviating severe headache pain. This process is only temporary and rarely will be effective in the long term; however, this technique is extremely effective for alleviating pain in the short term—perhaps late at night, early in the morning, after physician office hours, or while trying other treatments that may produce a more long-term and long-lasting pain relief effect.

Jane S. contacted Dr. Sudderth late one night, complaining of severe intractable headache pain associated with nausea. She did have anti-nausea medicine at home, but had no pain pills or other treatment regimen available. Rather than referring her to the emergency room for a pain shot, she was instructed to use ice therapy in the form of an ice pack at the base of her head for 20 minutes on, then 20 minutes off. She was to repeat this cycle over the next two to three hours, until she could be seen in the office early in the morning. Jane S. sounded disgusted, as though she felt she received no true therapeutic intervention. However, when she came in the next morning, she was delighted that the ice-pack therapy had indeed temporized her headache pain and alleviated her symptoms so she could relax. Once the anxiety over her migraine syndrome abated, she realized cryotherapy was truly effective in the short term.

Additional treatment intervention was discussed at the office visit, and ultimately the patient was able to abort her migraine, which she usually experienced as a cluster migraine that lasted three to four days. She was delighted she could stave off the onset of her severe cluster migraine with a treatment she could use independently, without medications or a trip to the Emergency Room.

HEAT THERAPY

The application of heat is an effective treatment for multiple processes, not just for headache pain. Heat is also quite effective for joint and arthritis pain. Anyone who walks down the pharmacy aisle can see that there is an enormous market for heating rubs and creams. If you watch enough television, you're sure to see at least one commercial espousing the virtues of deep heat and heating therapy to reduce pain.

The concept behind heat therapy is that heat opens the blood vessels, causing metabolic irritants to be carried away. It also allow enriched-oxygen-carrying blood cells to be transported to the inflamed area, thus nourishing and improving the inflamed area. Ultimately, this leads to tissue healing.

Heat also tends to increase the elasticity and flexibility of inflamed joints, tendons, and ligaments. This can be quite helpful in patients suffering from mixed headache disorders, who often have muscle tightness (contraction) in the head and neck.

Moist heat—applied through special heating pads, hot showers, and whirlpool baths—tends to be more effective than the dry heat obtained from a store-bought heating pad. Often, the moist heat application is performed for 20 to 40 minutes.

In general, heat therapy is relatively safe, effective, and inexpensive as a treatment option for patients suffering from occipital pain, head pain, craniofacial pain, and migraine. We feel that heat therapy works better for chronic pain than for an acute attack. In fact, once the acute attack has its onset, applying heating pads or other heat treatments to the base of the skull or neck may actually aggravate the migraine syndrome. Because this may lead to additional vasospasm (engorgement), it is not recommended. Indeed, as mentioned above, we use ice therapy at the onset, to temporize acute headache pains.

We do urge caution: Intense heat applied for prolonged periods of time can lead to a heat burn in certain individuals; therefore, we recommend common sense, good judgment, and appropriate treatment in the use of heat therapy.

HOMEOPATHIC MEDICATIONS AND REMEDIES

Today you can find homeopathic medications sold without a prescription in many pharmacies. Are they any good? Is there any validity to homeopathy?

While we consider ourselves traditional or "allopathic" physicians, we believe there are some important homeopathic interventions that are available, and we are aware that there is a great deal of value to some of these therapies.

Homeopathy, a discipline of nontraditional medicine, was founded by a German physician, Dr. Samuel Christian

Frederick Hahnemann, in the late eighteenth century. The term comes from the Greek word *homeo* (meaning similar) and *pathos* (meaning suffering from disease). In the simplest explanation, homeopathy is the practice of medicine in which "like cures like." The belief is that certain naturally occurring chemicals and processes that can produce symptoms in healthy people can, in low doses, cure those same symptoms in people suffering from illness. As noted, homeopathy has been present since the late 1700s, and clearly has provided some significant intervention in the role of pain management for migraine sufferers. Homeopathy is quite popular in many countries and cultures, and has slowly and steadily gained credibility and popularity in the United States.

If traditional medicine were to produce cures in all patients, then homeopathy would have fallen out of favor. At the same time, if homeopathic medicine provided all the answers, then we would not have traditional physicians and neurologists who are actively seeking to provide pain relief to migraineurs.

How does homeopathic medicine work—if it does work? The concept is that a minute dose of a substance that would be harmful in high doses can stimulate healing in the body. For example, belladonna is a deadly poison when a large enough dose is taken. In very small doses, it may actually cure your migraine. Homeopathic medicine may allow the body to heal itself by "resetting" the body's imbalances that led to the migraine headache. How it does this remains a mystery to us.

A variety of chemicals and medications are popular among homeopathic physicians. Each one appears to direct its action against specific symptoms. Remember that patients respond differently to different medications. This is also true with homeopathic medicine. Just because a medication is not "prescription" does not mean it is entirely safe, benign, or usable in an unlimited and unrestricted fashion.

As a result, it is important to practice a trial approach to homeopathic medicines (under the guidance of the expert), just as you would with traditional medicines.

Belladonna seems to be effective for patients who have severe intractable headaches that are associated with throbbing blood vessels and facial flushing, as well as with headaches aggravated by standing and improved by sitting down.

Bryonia seems to work with motion-sensitive headaches, as well as headaches associated with moderate pain behind the eyes. In addition, migraines that are present in the early morning, particularly upon awakening, may respond to bryonia. If you feel sinus congestion or fullness, you may have a positive response to this agent.

Nux vomica, another homeopathic remedy, may bring some relief if your migraines appear to be induced by eating or drinking, such as consuming coffee or another caffeinated substance. In addition, if basic sleep, nutrition, diet, or activity level changes trigger your migraine, you may respond to *nux vomica.*

Pulsatilla is a substance that may help if you are suffering from the "brain freeze" of eating a cold substance that triggers the migraine. If smoking or overindulging in rich foods causes your migraine, you may also be a responder.

Gelsemium is another homeopathic remedy; it seems most effective if your headache syndrome begins at the back of your neck and radiates forward. Headaches associated with a visual aura may also respond to this treatment.

Sanguinaria is a homeopathic remedy for patients who suffer from migraine pain on one side of the head. Also, intractable headaches without pounding and throbbing may respond to this treatment.

Some herbs may be used to treat migraine headaches. For example, feverfew seems fairly effective for some patients as a preventive measure to avoid the acute migraine episode. Articles reviewed by the National Headache Foundation have stated that feverfew is somewhat effective for migraine prevention. Apparently, this herb must be taken on a regular basis. It should be noted that feverfew use is still considered experimental therapy among traditional neurologists in the

United States. It is, however, among the most commonly prescribed medications in England, having shown great success for migraine headache control in that population.

We suggest that those interested in more information about homeopathic medicines, herbal treatments, herbology, and additional botanicals and natural pharmaceuticals do a more extensive review of the available literature. It is interesting to note that many current prescription medicines have their origin or basis in natural herbal/plant origin, but have been produced in a synthetic fashion to simulate natural treatments.

As we have suggested, a combined approach to pain management is often the best approach. Combining therapeutic regimens, including natural treatments, cryotherapy or diathermy, exercise or breathing, or any other relaxation techniques can also provide you with a powerful and complete "toolbox" to treat your migraine pain syndrome. Because many of these therapeutic and relaxation interventions require practice, we suggest that people train in these modalities prior to an acute attack. The rewards of mastering these techniques can be immense, not only in migraine pain management, but also in the general sense of wellness and well-being. These techniques can empower you to overcome your headache pain syndrome, as well as lead a more relaxed, stress-free, and enriched life.

In the next chapter, we discuss yet another form of natural intervention: biofeedback therapy. This has actually gained significant credibility among traditional physicians, and has been touted by the National Headache Foundation as an ideal treatment, at times the first-time treatment for tension and muscle contraction headaches. This rediscovered technique and therapy regimen is now used in a number of settings, providing physicians and patients with yet another powerful tool in the battle against migraine headache pain.

12

BIOFEEDBACK

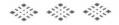

What would you say if we told you a therapy is available that will help you prevent and treat migraines as well as daily headaches, and improve the way in which your body responds to stress—one that is cheap, easy on your liver, and keeps right on working?

Well, such a therapy is very easy to access. Why then don't you know about this remarkable option? Is it a right- or left-wing conspiracy, or just those evil drug companies wanting you to take their medications by the supertankerful? Probably none of the above. Exercise and weight loss will make us look and feel better and add about a decade to our lives. Why then don't we heed that mountain of medical evidence? Because it takes time, effort, and practice. And so does the single, most effective, nonpharmacological treatment for migraine: biofeedback.

Biofeedback is a conditioning regimen that allows the patient to learn to control physiologic functions that are not typically under voluntary control. A short list of examples would include skin temperature, muscle tension in various sites, heart rate, blood pressure, and even brain electrical activity. Conventional biofeedback (CBF) concerns itself primarily with heart rate, skin temperature, and muscle tension (contraction). A relative newcomer to the scene is neurofeedback, in which brain wave frequencies are the object of the conditioning procedure. We will consider conventional biofeedback first.

As we mentioned, biofeedback involves the influence, if not mastery over certain physiologic functions, most of which are traditionally described as "autonomic functions." This refers to the autonomic nervous system, which normally goes about its business without your telling it what to do. The autonomic system deals primarily with digestion, elimination, and sexual function, but appears also to be intimately involved in pain sensation. Divided into the sympathetic and parasympathetic portions, the autonomic nervous system wields an iron hand over our comfort and bodily ("vegetative") functions. The sympathetic symptoms ready us to stand our ground or run in the face of a perceived threat (fight or flight). At one time this response was helpful to our survival. The sympathetic nervous system allows us to send blood to the brain and muscles that need increased energy and oxygen during this response, and away from skin, intestine, and genitals. The heart rate and blood pressure increase to maintain the metabolic requirements for dealing with the threat in question. This is also when the sweating and heavy breathing starts. This is all well and good as long as the threat is a genuine danger to our survival, but can lead to a problem if the threat is the boss' bad mood or concern about making a traffic light!

Thus, we see that many of the symptoms of migraine appear to be related to the autonomic nervous system. Pallor, nausea, pain, lightheadedness, swelling, and irritability are, at least in part, autonomic mediated. Does this mean that migraine is a pure autonomic disruption? Probably not. However, there is evidence to suggest that the autonomic nervous system is disordered in individuals with migraine. In an article recently published in the prestigious journal,

Headache (39:108–117, 1999), Dr. Amnon Mosek suggests that the autonomic nervous system, particularly the sympathetic system, is dysfunctional in individuals with migraine, particularly migraine with aura. Dr. Mosek has demonstrated abnormalities in the maintenance of blood pressure under various conditions, while other researchers have demonstrated abnormalities in other aspects of the autonomic nervous system in individuals suffering from migraine.

If you are interested in trying biofeedback, discuss this therapy with your physician. Most physicians are aware of biofeedback as a treatment option for migraine and headaches in general and will gladly refer you for training. Typically, the therapy will be done at a hospital, free-standing physical therapy center, or in the physician's office. Recently, many chiropractors have begun offering biofeedback, a practice we welcome. Conventional biofeedback does not appear to have any negative side effects. However, we recommend that patients consult their physician since migraine and other headache-type symptoms can relate to other conditions requiring further diagnostic studies and/or therapy. We are well aware that biofeedback home units are readily available over the Internet and other sources. While these instruments may be beneficial for some individuals, we recommend that the therapy be initiated under the watchful eye of your physician.

The two types of biofeedback training typically offered will be discussed below: thermal biofeedback (blood flow) or electromyographic (EMG).

Thermal Biofeedback

This is the most commonly used type of conventional biofeedback for individuals suffering from migraine. The patient learns to increase the blood flow and consequently the temperature on the fingers. A small temperature-recording device (thermistor) is attached to a finger. It relays the information to a computer, which will then display the temperature in a graphic mode on the monitor. The patient is instructed, "Warm your fingers." As this occurs, changes on the monitor will indicate increased blood flow to the fingers. Although the patient will not be successful immediately, after many sessions he or she will be able to increase the blood flow significantly and consistently in the fingers. The subject is encouraged to practice this not only inside but outside the training facility. Increasing this type of control over the cardiovascular system appears to be effective in not only treating headaches but also in preventing them.

Electromyographic (EMG) Biofeedback

In this type of therapy, the raw data is supplied by electrodes overlying the skin over various muscles. Typically, these will be about the face, neck, and head. While most skeletal muscles are under voluntary control, at certain sites voluntary muscle seems to have a will of its own. This is particularly true in the muscles of the face, the trapezius, and the chewing muscles. Data from the electrodes indicating the amount of spontaneous muscular activity will be conveyed via the computer monitor to the patient, who will be rewarded by graphic or audio feedback as the muscle activity decreases. This sounds very simple but typically requires several visits to master.

Does Biofeedback Really Work?

The answer to this question is only maybe. Not everyone benefits from this type of therapy in terms of headache relief, although the literature suggest that at least half the individuals who master the conditioning techniques will improve in terms of their headaches. The individuals may not be able to entirely withdraw all their medications, but most patients will have less need for migraine medications. The ability to control the "flight or fight response" can be generalized outside the laboratory and can have a profound impact on the patient's life overall. This type of therapy is a very potent stress buster and can be combined with a great benefit with other types of therapy such as relaxation therapy and cognitive therapy.

While biofeedback can be effective for anyone suffering from headaches or migraine in particular, it is especially viable in certain patient populations, and is quite accessible and inexpensive. Unfortunately, it is not covered by all private insurance or by Medicare. No adverse side effects are known to occur with this type of therapy.

This is clearly a first-line therapy for pregnant women. Women who are pregnant or lactating will not have to worry about possible fetal complications. It is particularly important for the child-bearing age group to avoid medication that may have a profound but as yet unrecognized impact. In addition, many recent studies have demonstrated how sensitive older adults are to medications. A recent publication even suggested that improper use of prescription medications may be a common cause of death in senior citizens. Although those in the older population group do not appear to learn techniques such as biofeedback as quickly as do those in other age groups, they too can master these techniques given appropriate training. For this reason, we ardently hope that Medicare will cover this type of therapy in the future.

There are certain obstacles to effective biofeedback training. Many patients have difficulty believing that nonpharmacological therapy can have such a powerful and generalized effect on the migraine sufferer's life. This issue is best dealt with by the referring physician explaining the therapy in some detail. A qualified biofeedback technician can also be helpful in this regard. Individuals on large quantities of pain relievers may not benefit from biofeedback therapy. These patients often must be detoxified, possibly on an in-patient basis, prior to beginning treatment.

We have used biofeedback effectively in our practice for about ten years. Approximately 70% of patients suffering from migraine symptoms find some relief in severity, duration, and frequency of their migraines. All our patients who have completed a course of biofeedback endorse this technology as a powerful, life-changing experience.

It is clear from the literature, however, that conventional biofeedback does not help everyone. Still, we feel that this technology is greatly underutilized and should be started early in the therapeutic regimen in any individual suffering from migraine.

Neurofeedback (NF)

In neurofeedback (NF), peripheral parameters such as skin temperature and muscle contraction are no longer the primary focus for conditioning. In NF the therapist goes right to where the money is in migraine: to the brain itself. This exciting technology has been available for over 20 years but has only recently become a viable treatment modality posting great success in many conditions such as anxiety, chronic pain, epilepsy, and attention deficit disorder (to name only a few).

Central to NF is the electroencephalogram (EEG), the development of which is credited to the German researcher Hans Berger in 1920. The EEG records tiny waves of brain activity over the scalp with the help of very small electrodes. This technique has evolved into a powerful diagnostic tool in modern medicine, assisting the physician in the evaluation of epilepsy, dementia, and coma. While traditional EEG has not been helpful in the diagnosis of migraine per se, abnormalities in this examination have been reported by many researchers, who have found deviant electrical behavior in the brains of migraineurs both during and between migraine attacks. A cyber-era refinement of traditional EEG—quantitative EEG (QEEG)—is pushing this technology into a more intimate and fundamental study of normal and diseased brain activity.

Like the autonomic functions discussed above, the EEG has not been considered an area over which an individual could develop voluntary control—until now, that is! By being "fed back" brain wave data via analogous representations on a computer monitor, the individual can unconsciously train herself to control what she sees on the monitor. This type of training has been reported to significantly reduce the frequency of migraine attacks in selected individuals. While the supporting data at present are anecdotal, many researchers are currently at work establishing NF as a viable treatment option for migraine and other types of headache. The implications of this technology for both health and disease are far-reaching. We are convinced that NF is the most promising alternative therapy regimen in existence today.

13

TAKING CONTROL: LIFESTYLE CHANGES

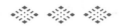

U p to this point, we have discussed migraine and other types of headaches, multiple facets relating to migraine disorders, and how physicians approach issues relating to diagnosing and treating migraineurs. Now we will focus on how *you* can take control of your activities and other aspects of your life to work toward preventing migraines from occurring, or at least minimizing the pain they cause. The following suggestions can also improve your overall physical functioning.

GETTING YOUR BODY INTO A HEALTHY CYCLE

Our bodies are complex machines, and just like other complicated pieces of equipment, they cannot be run 24 hours a day without some "down time." Also like intricate equipment, we need frequent maintenance and periodic checkups.

Most importantly of all, we function most efficiently when we are on a basic routine. The body works on a chemical routine, particularly with relation to the peaks and valleys related to the adrenaline chemicals that are produced. We have peaks of cortisol, an adrenaline chemical, at approximately 6:00 A.M. and 4:00 P.M. This may explain why we start out the day with energy, by early to mid-afternoon have periods of fatigue, then in late afternoon get a "second wind."

When we try to break this cycle or resist our bodies' natural rhythm, we can end up experiencing a general sense of fatigue, malaise, and being unwell. As mentioned previously, any illness and any competition with our bodies' natural rhythms can certainly act as a migraine or headache trigger. Therefore, it is best to pick a routine and try to regiment our lifestyle enough so that we can live comfortably within the boundaries of our routine.

This is not to say that we expect our readers to become robots with a rigidly restricted lifestyle, looking at the clock every hour to maintain their regimen. Rather, we recommend that you try to wake up at the same time every morning and eat three to four small, well-balanced meals per day. Space out work and exercise, as well as your social obligations and stressful activities, in a pattern comfortable for you.

We know this can't always be done. Maybe your mother-in-law or boss is coming for dinner, the kids just came down with chicken pox, and you're also juggling a difficult project—so for today you have to throw out most of your schedule. These things happen. But within the parameters of your life, you do have quite a bit of control (yes, you do!), and we want you to use it.

Everyone needs to examine his or her lifestyle to determine what the daily priorities are and to then determine how those can be broken up. One of the common factors in patients who experience migraines when they travel is the fact that they are not only having altitude and geographic changes, but also changes to their daily routine. We frequently hear "My whole vacation was ruined by my migraine headaches."

Part of this is because you may be consuming foods different from your usual diet. But a bigger part of the problem is that you may get yourself completely out of sync; for example, a time zone change can throw you off because it affects your sleeping and eating patterns, and there also may be climactic and altitude changes, as well as other differences from your normal life.

We recommend to our patients that even when they travel, they try to maintain a routine lifestyle, or at least as close to a routine lifestyle as possible.

Pearl of wisdom: As we mentioned earlier in this chapter, our cortisol level drops early in the afternoon, and doesn't pick up again until late afternoon. This may explain why most country's citizens (with the notable exception of people in the United States) take naps or respite periods after lunchtime.

Although you may not be able to take an afternoon nap, it may still be a good idea to avoid over-exerting yourself in the mid-afternoon, particularly if you are prone to peaks and valleys of adrenaline chemicals in your body.

SLEEP BETTER, LIVE BETTER

Following through on this concept of a routine lifestyle, we certainly cannot ignore what for most people is approximately one-third of their life—sleep time. We have often heard the expression, "If I could just get a good night's sleep, I know I would feel better." This is absolutely true. Sleep is an important physiological function that acts to restore the body's nutrients and indeed allows us to "re-set the computer."

When we have difficulties with sleep initiation (insomnia), as well as difficulties with staying asleep or waking up too early, we often do not fully recharge our bodies. In this sense, we're much like a nickel cadmium rechargeable battery. If the body is not drained down completely, then when it is charged, the charge does not last as long. Certainly, if we do not get a full complement or battery of sleep, when we do awaken, we are rarely as refreshed or energetic as we would like to be, nor do we "last as long" without becoming fatigued and sleepy.

The American Sleep Disorders Foundation has eloquently stated that many actually acquire a "sleep debt." People will go for days or even weeks getting too little sleep and then have to spend a few days actually replacing that sleep debt with a long weekend of extended sleep pattern.

Certainly, this extreme variation in the day/night cycle, and in the body's natural rhythms, can lead to discomfort and can even be a potent trigger for illness, including migraines.

Correcting the Sleep Problem

It is clear that before we can correct the sleep problem, we need to identify what is actually causing the sleep disturbance. For many individuals, it is the chemicals that they ingest, but for others it is lifestyle stressors, inappropriate activities, or simply an uncomfortable sleeping environment.

Indeed, one of the most notorious triggers for insomnia is actually sleep medications. While they may work for a series of days, they frequently lead to a rebound phenomenon, a secondary insomnia, which is quite difficult to treat.

Specialists who deal with sleep disorders often recommend a comprehensive sleep evaluation, even going so far as monitoring someone's sleep in a laboratory at nighttime. If there is a reversal of one's day/night cycle, or if someone is off by "two or three hours" after traveling, many techniques can be used to "re-set your time clock"; however, these are not trivial and are best discussed with a specialist in sleep disorders.

To correct a problematic sleep cycle, follow these simple rules:

- Do not consume any caffeine or stimulant medication close to bedtime. Many authorities would recommend avoiding caffeine entirely at any time, particularly if there is any sleep problem, and certainly if caffeine is a headache trigger for you.

- Avoid alcoholic beverages prior to bedtime. The idea of "just a nightcap will help me fall asleep" may be correct, but almost assuredly will wake you up within a few hours.

Actually, alcohol does three things to the central nervous system: irritates, inflames, and depresses. So while alcohol may act as a central nervous system depressant initially, there is a profound rebound effect that occurs within two to three hours and also acts as a rebound stimulant.

This is why individuals who imbibe alcoholic beverages in mid-evening can often be drowsy throughout the night but later on are "wide awake and ready to keep going."

- If you cannot sleep, it is absolutely essential that you get up, get out of bed, and do something else. Do not lie in bed and wait for sleep to come; oftentimes it will not, and trying to sleep just leads to a frustration or anxiety situation, which then leads to additional sleep dysfunction.

- Avoid re-setting the "sleep clock" by taking little naps throughout the course of the day. We do allow some of our senior citizens to take a one-half to one-hour nap after lunch, when the cortisol levels are low, but this would be only if their naps do not compromise their sleep habits (i.e., keep them up later than usual). With regard to our migraine sufferers, we absolutely do not want them to interrupt their day cycle with sleep, as that will also interrupt their night cycle with wakefulness.

- Do not go to bed angry or stressed. While this sounds simple, it is surprising how many people will truly "take their problems to bed," and then simply rehash them all night. They toss and turn, which clearly is unhealthy.

We explain to our patients that it is very important they resolve their crises, problems, or dilemmas prior to sleep. Yes, we know this is easy to say, hard to do. But try it! It has worked for many. Despite sounding simple and trivial, our patients have told us that when they do follow this instruction, they have a much more restful night of sleep.

Now that we have discussed what not to do, we can be more positive by pointing out actions that are helpful when you want to fall to sleep.

- Work on, practice, and develop positive relaxation techniques to initiate drowsiness and restfulness.

- Be assertive—prepare your sleep environment to make it comfortable for you. Specifically, eliminate activity, noises, sounds, or lights that keep you awake. Many individuals tell us that with "white noise," or soothing background noise, they can effectively block out irritating noise.

- Check with your doctor and check with your pharmacist for guidance. Frequently, even medications that have been taken for a long period of time, or medicines that your physician has told you "won't have any side effects," may in fact have a stimulant effect. It is important to check on this, as there is almost always more than one medication for any one illness.

Don't be afraid to communicate with your physician that this disruption in your sleep cycle is an issue. It certainly is an issue when you suffer from migraine headache disorder.

In addition to those general concepts for preparing for a proper sleep cycle, some more specific suggestions are often helpful. For example, L-tryptophan, an amino acid, has been noted to be quite helpful for sleep initiation. This drug was recently banned from the United States, but is once again available here as well as in other countries. However, there are also many natural methods of obtaining L-tryptophan.

Foods high in L-tryptophan content include such things as bananas, yogurt, dates, and milk. (See? Your mom was right if she told you to drink a nice glass of milk before bed!)

In addition, certain vitamins and supplements have also been found somewhat helpful in improving sleep initiation, such as Vitamin B3, as well as calcium and magnesium. Indeed, numerous investigations currently underway have revealed that magnesium is a potent mineral and may play an extremely important role in aborting acute migraine headaches.

Also, many herbs are helpful for sleep initiation, such as valerian root and passion flower.

Leg Cramp Problems

We are frequently questioned about nighttime leg cramps, which often awaken patients from sleep and seem to prevent the re-initiation of sleep. Prescription medications such as quinine sulfate and Quinam can help alleviate this problem. But a more natural approach can include such simple measures as good relaxation techniques prior to bed, as well as taking Vitamin E supplements. We have had quite good results with this.

Natural Sleep Substance

Lastly, a natural hormone, melatonin, reaches its peak of activity during sleep. Produced in the pineal gland, melatonin seems to play a powerful role in maintaining a regular hormonal and circadian cycle (a daily fluctuation of hormone release and other physiological functions). At the present time, prescription melatonin is not widely available. For more information regarding how to obtain this chemical, see listings under Important National Organizations, in the Appendix.

EXERCISE

If you look around at the newspaper, on television, or at your local bookstore, you will gain the impression that exercise is a cure for everything, or at least that seems to be what people want you to believe. And they are probably right. Not only does exercise help you look good, it actually enables you to feel good and be well.

A number of processes occur with routine exercise, such as increasing your metabolism, burning fat, reducing calories, and improving your cardiovascular system. For patients suffering from migraine disorders, routine exercise can actually produce complex chemical changes in the brain that may ward off future migraine attacks.

We have one patient who tells us that when he gets his migraine headaches, he will actually "go for a jog" to try to avoid a severe attack from coming on. Often his migraine episode is completely aborted within 5 to 10 minutes, without any of the severe nausea or secondary phenomenon.

How does this work? Well, we think that the exercise-induced chemical change induces a blockade of chemical response, thereby preventing the blood vessels going in and out of spasm, and reducing the ultimate pounding, throbbing, and pulsing headache pain.

To provide an example, the exercise produces chemical messengers that act sort of as a key fitting into the lock. When these chemical messengers (the good guys) fit in the lock, that means that the poisons or toxins that occur at the time of a migraine headache cannot fit into this same "lock."

Therefore, the whole cascade effect (discussed in chapter 2: Theories of Migraine) cannot occur, and we are "protected." While exercise does not produce this effect in every individual, certainly it has many benefits for virtually everyone.

We often recommend that patients do a combination of exercise, not just body toning or just aerobic activity. We combine a low-impact aerobic program with a weight or resistance training program, in combination with proper body mechanics (to be discussed later).

We generally recommend 30 to 40 minutes of aerobic activities three to four times per week plus a resistance training program with low weights and multiple repetitions three to four times a week for 30 to 40 minutes each.

We know what you are thinking—we've heard it before. "But Doctor, I don't *have* 60 to 80 minutes a day to exercise!" However, when you think about it, if you provide yourself with positive reinforcement and positive conditioning by training for approximately one hour per day, that still leaves 23 hours in your whole day. This seems a pretty reasonable balance when you consider that the return can be a pain-free existence.

NUTRITION: "YOU ARE WHAT YOU EAT"

Most of us have automobiles or often ride in automobiles. If you have ever obtained bad gasoline, you know what the effect can be. Your car does not run well, and ultimately you suffer for it. The initial savings the cheaper gasoline may have offered is far outweighed by the frustration, annoyance, and ultimately larger costs one has to pay down the road.

Our bodies also require good fuel to run well. While neither of us is extremist about diet or habits, we do promote the values of moderation, particularly when it comes to a proper diet. And for migraine sufferers, a proper diet can be everything.

In the 1960s, the rage was for neurologists to place patients on what is called an "oligo-antigenic diet." This is a special type of elimination diet. It allows the dieter to pinpoint what foods may be migraine triggers by introducing food back into the diet one type at a time. We have come a long way since this diet, yet as we have discussed in our chapter on food fright, diet is still absolutely essential in managing the migraine headache.

It isn't possible to know every ingredient in each food, but certainly reading labels is appropriate, as is avoiding toxins such as caffeine (found in beverages such as coffee, tea, and colas as well as foods made from cocoa), avoiding processed foods high in sulfites or MSG, and staying away from foods containing excessive yeast, nitrates/nitrites, or tyramine.

Although a glass of milk may help you get to sleep, for some migraineurs, dairy products can have a negative impact. This fact is certainly outlined in the National Headache Foundation's Diet, as well as in numerous additional diets for migraine patients.

So what type of diet is an appropriate diet to prevent or control migraine attacks? Experts disagree, but we feel the key is moderation. While in some instances it is a good idea to go to a complete elimination diet, introducing one food at a time, it certainly is reasonable to cut down on foods high in cholesterol, fat, and sugar content.

In addition, too much red meat may act as a food trigger, thus your intake of red meat certainly should be reduced. Since red meat is predominantly made up of fat and protein, too much red meat may in turn lead to a high protein count, which then has to be metabolized. Physicians have already found that in certain illnesses such as liver and kidney disease, as well as in neurologic illness such as Parkinson's, a low-protein diet can be very effective in controlling them. Certainly, many theories regarding low-protein diets have also been hypothesized for migraine disorders.

In addition, it is reasonable to consider a routine daily multivitamin/multimineral supplement. However, we urge you away from a mega-vitamin preparation. In addition, avoid the "amino acid therapy," which we see many of today's teens using, particularly teenage athletes.

There are good vitamins that are effective as anti-oxidants, a topic which certainly has received some popular press over the last few years. Such chemicals include Vitamins E and C, selenium, and even beta-carotene. You can go to any health food store and find a wide variety and complement of combinations of these antioxidants, as well as of vitamin and mineral supplements. (The Life Guide Diet Supplement, which is listed in the Appendix, is an example of a vitamin preparation.)

When patients come to us with migraine disorders, we ask that they bring all the chemicals and medicines they take, including natural treatments, non-prescription medications, and over-the-counter medications. It is surprising what patients will take in the name of "natural herbs and supplements," just because it does not require a prescription from a physician.

Additional supplements that are often found in good multi-vitamin/multimineral supplements include chromium, copper, iron, manganese, molybdenum, potassium, and zinc.

Key Supplements

While Vitamin B6 (pyridoxine) may not be the one essential ingredient for a neurochemical process, it is now recognized as a powerful cofactor for almost every neurologic chemical process that occurs in the body.

Specifically, one can think of B6 as a taxi driver for additional chemicals and nutrients. B6 helps the chemicals and nutrients get where they need to be, but does not actually participate in the chemical reaction once these materials reach their destination.

Much like the taxi driver, B6 is a cofactor and is extremely important. In neurology, we see B6 deficiency producing seizures, particularly in children and newborn infants. A B6 deficiency also plays a significant role in headache disorder, particularly vascular headaches.

Other complications of B6 deficiency include neuropathy (nerve damage in the extremities), behavior change, mood swings, depression, and even movement disorders. B6 deficiency can actually have a significant role in perpetuating a chronic pain syndrome.

In addition, a subset of migraine exists that occurs with the chemical and hormonal shifts associated with premenstrual syndrome, which is quite well addressed with a combined effect of pyridoxine (B6) and magnesium.

As mentioned, B6 seems to be an important chemical link for many chemical reactions in the body, particularly as the "express taxi driver" for magnesium. Recently magnesium has received a lot of attention with regard to numerous medical processes, including providing significant relief for migraine headaches.

Magnesium

While we are talking about supplements, we should spend a moment discussing the positive breakthroughs with regard to understanding the role of magnesium. We now know that a lack of magnesium in the diet can lead to deficiencies, but we also know that other medical illnesses, including sugar diabetes, thyroid disease, and multiple medications, can lead to this deficiency of magnesium as well.

Alcohol and prolonged stress can also be factors in a low magnesium level. In addition to triggering a migraine headache or promoting a migraine into a severe sick headache, symptoms of low magnesium can include muscle cramps, general fatigue, sleep disturbance, irritability, and muscle tension.

As mentioned earlier, prolonged stress or illness can lead to a magnesium deficiency. Here we see a cyclical pattern, that the low magnesium level leads to illness, and the illness continues the low magnesium level by depleting magnesium stores.

We recommend to our patients that they have their magnesium levels monitored, and we also recommend that magnesium-deficient patients may increase their magnesium levels through consuming such foods as nuts, beans, whole grains, and fish.

Because the magnesium seems to play a significant role in stabilizing the blood vessel walls, thus preventing the spasm, it is absolutely critical that physicians take a look at magnesium levels. While it is unlikely that magnesium is the sole culprit in causing or allowing a migraine to continue, it is nevertheless an easily and quickly treated problem, and therefore should be addressed and remedied.

We strongly recommend that you discuss vitamin deficiencies and whether you should take a general vitamin and mineral supplement with your physician to make sure you are on the right path with regard to overall nutritional wellness. One popular and relatively complete supplement is the Life Guide Adult Daily Dietary Supplement, which can be obtained at many natural health stores. (More information on this supplement is included in the Appendix.)

Herbs and Natural Ingredients

While traditional Western medicine places great stock in the value of prescription medications, it is important to realize that almost every medication has its origins in a natural product, almost always plant products.

Keeping this in mind, you shouldn't be surprised that a natural alternative to prescription medications are herbs, which may be used as medicinal agents. There are literally thousands of these available at the natural health stores, and one has to exercise great judgment and caution in approaching them, just as you should with any over-the-counter medicine or any prescription medicine.

As we tell our patients, any chemical can have any reaction in any one individual, so it is important to make sure that you know what the potential desired effect is, and then monitor for side effects appropriately.

In previous chapters, we have discussed a handful of natural ingredients that are frequently used to treat migraine pain. Another common example is feverfew. This member of the daisy family is believed to work by blocking serotonin release. Also, it possibly inhibits the release of additional chemical substances in the brain that are responsible for causing the spasm in the blood vessel walls. This is an extremely popular chemical remedy in England.

Additional herbal treatments for acute migraine attacks include white willow bark, a compound very similar to aspirin. Also, L-tryptophan used as an amino acid supplement may actually help raise the pain threshold, thereby reducing the appreciation of pain. An additional amino acid, phenylalanine, may actually be able to block the breakdown of the brain's natural pain medicines, endorphins/enkephalins. Endorphins, which are the chemical released to produce the "runner's high" in long distance runners, are much like morphine, and can be used as natural painkillers.

Since literally hundreds of chemicals are available for the natural treatment of pain and migraines, we refer you to our list of resources in the Appendix on where to obtain more information.

Posture

Parents often say: "Sit up straight, keep your back straight, don't slouch." Once again, Mom (or Dad) was right. Posture plays a significant role in maintaining proper spine alignment and preventing the forces of injury, which can lead to muscle spasm and muscle contraction. As we have discussed, there are multiple theories of migraine, yet the brain itself does not appreciate pain. There are no pain-sensitive structures in the brain. We experience pain from either involvement of the arteries and small arterioles, or from the sensation triggers in the neck, head, and joints.

When we slouch, stoop forward, hold our head in one isolated posture for prolonged periods of time, we have improper forces applied to the cervical musculature, and with this there is tension and stress on the supporting structures of the head and neck. This then leads to spasm, waste products from the spasm, including toxins, and ultimately, spasm of the blood vessels. Along with these actions, there is also a decreased circulation, decreased oxygen and nutrition, and ultimately, we experience pain.

We recommend that our patients follow proper body mechanics (please see neck exercises in the Appendix) and make frequent changes in position. Don't keep your head or neck in any isolated posture for more than 40 to 45 minutes at a time without a 3 to 5 minute change in position.

While this may sound like a significant time commitment, especially in a work environment with close supervision, one can take a 3 to 5 minute change in position by changing from the computer to do filing, from filing to walking to the water cooler or copier, and so on. As a result, we don't mean that you have to put a screeching halt to all activity every 45 minutes. It merely means you should change positions.

It's also important to note that individuals who follow a routine exercise regimen, utilize proper body mechanics, and demonstrate good posture, rarely will have the secondary muscle contraction phenomenon that seems to plague many migraine sufferers. Migraineurs may develop a mixed headache disorder, having both migraines and their daily headache pains, which are not true migraines. Because proper body posture can eliminate secondary muscle contraction, we outline key ways to achieve good posture in our Appendix under Activities for Daily Living. Proper stretching and flexibility exercises are also presented.

DEFICIENCY IN THE "COPING CHROMOSOME"

We all have our own ways to handle both physical and emotional stress. Some people ignore the problem; others tackle it head-on. Some internalize problems, while others verbalize them until everyone knows about their situation. With migraine pain, the most important thing is to enhance your own personal coping mechanisms.

We do not have a "coping chromosome." Instead, we learn through our environment, society, and positive and negative reinforcements on how to deal effectively with stressful situations.

Certainly, recurrent headaches, as well as intractable migraines, can be considered both an external and internal stress. We need to not only alleviate the pain, but improve our outlook and reduce the anxiety that comes with the expectation of pain. We need to regain control of our lives.

But how? One of the first things that we instruct our patients to do is to identify triggers and eliminate these from their environment. Specifically, you are to avoid chemicals, toxins, and body pollutants (tobacco, alcohol, caffeine, etc.) you are currently using. In fact, it is important you remove these triggers from your environment altogether if possible.

If your spouse smokes, make it clear that their smoke may be triggering your headache pains; therefore, this situation needs to be remedied. If your spouse is unable or unwilling to give up smoking, could he or she confine the smoking to an outside area? Can you seek other mutually acceptable solutions?

In addition, make sure you follow a good lifestyle regimen, which includes frequent nutritional meals and avoidance of low sugar (hypoglycemic) states.

How you perceive your pain is another important issue you need to address. If, with the onset of a mild, dull headache you become anxious and your heart races, you become fearful that maybe you'll develop a severe migraine. Often this reaction itself will promote the very reactions you want so badly to avoid.

Using the nonpharmacologic treatments listed in other chapters, you can often immediately perform one or more of these activities (muscle relaxation, deep breathing, guided imagery, etc.) to help block the secondary response to migraine. Yes, a dull headache may present and may progress into a migraine. Yet how we react to this and how we interact immediately plays a significant role in determining what our ultimate level of illness and dysfunction may be.

We have one patient who explained to us that when he feels his headache coming on, he steps into the bathroom and uses an Imitrex injection. He will remain in the toilet stall for 8 to 12 minutes. The result is that nearly every single sequential event leading up to the migraine has been completely aborted, with the patient able to resume unrestricted work activities. In the meantime, not a single co-employee knew that he had a severe headache/migraine, nor does anyone notice those few minutes away from his work station. As a result, this migraineur has had no negative repercussions, and has been a very successful employee.

Many of our patients have complained of a multitude of psychological symptoms, either directly or indirectly associated with their migraine headaches: fatigue, sadness, depression, crying spells, feelings of emptiness and hopelessness, anxiety, and especially a "generalized or free-floating anxiety." Patients also complain of an overall lack of drive, lack of appetite, decreased attention and concentration, and memory disturbances.

It is essential to be able to identify these sensations as they correlate with migraine headache pain. It is equally critical to take control of these feelings, emotions, and attitudes in order to effect a positive response to your headache treatment, and also to your lifestyle and general sense of wellness.

Sometimes, however, you may need assistance from a mental professional who can help you develop additional coping mechanisms and undergo personal growth counseling. You may need an unbiased, objective listener who can see aspects of your lifestyle or behaviors that you yourself can't see (just as you couldn't see the "Kick Me!" sign another third grader taped to your back) and who can play a role in your recovery. An unbiased professional may be able to determine other triggers, other activities in which you are engaging that somehow may be promoting your migraine headaches. In addition, the mental health professional may be able to identify associated psychological symptoms that come on with the anxiety and stress of a headache syndrome.

As you can see, it is important to follow a complete lifestyle approach to headache pain management, which includes avoidance of inappropriate medication, herbs, or chemicals; replacement of the proper body minerals, nutrients, and vitamin supplements; diet; exercise; and proper body mechanics. A proper sleep and life cycle and a positive outlook can all play a tremendous role in improving your headache syndrome and alleviating your migraine dysfunction.

Remember, the migraines did not come on overnight, and certainly a lifestyle approach can lead to a lifetime cure. The rewards of a headache-free existence make it worth any inconvenience at first to establish an appropriate lifestyle for preventing future migraine suffering.

14

Frequently Asked Questions

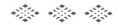

In this chapter, we include questions we are asked over and over—as well as a few unusual questions people have asked us.

QUESTION: *My headaches don't fall into any of the usual patterns. I have a headache almost every day and a sick headache two or three times monthly. I have a severe unilateral throbbing headache associated with intense nausea, vomiting, and increased sensitivity to light and sound. What kind of headache is this, and what do I do about it?*

ANSWER: It sounds like you have more than one type of headache. The daily headaches are probably related to muscle contraction, which is discussed elsewhere in the book. The more infrequent unilateral headaches certainly sound like migraines.

Individuals who suffer from migraines are frequently more prone to other types of headaches such as daily muscle contraction headaches. Some forms of therapy are good for both types of headaches—such as tricyclic medications or aspirin, as well as techniques resulting in stress reduction, while other types of therapy, such as ergotamine or Sumatriptan, would be specific for migraine.

QUESTION: *I have suffered from migraines for approximately ten years. Some medications such as Cafergot and Sumatriptan have been somewhat helpful with the acute attacks. However, I still suffer from migraines two to three times monthly and miss at least one day a month from work because of these headaches.*

I have tried propranolol, Elavil, Pamelor, Prozac, and two or three other medications that I cannot recall. Moreover, I have tried limiting various items from my diet without success.

I have also tried biofeedback, acupuncture, and even other less mainstream forms of therapy without success. What do I do now?

ANSWER: The most important thing for you is not to give up, but to continue to educate yourself about your condition. Frequently, changes in diet, activity, or a new medication overlooked previously can have a dramatic effect on the course and control of migraine therapy. Moreover, new therapies are constantly being added to our anti-migrainous arsenal. As with any chronic medical condition, a positive attitude and vigilance usually pay off in one way or another.

QUESTION: *I have had migraines since childhood. My headaches have been quite severe and have interfered with work as well as my life in general.*

My mother has headaches similar to mine, as does my only sister. My headaches have been such a nuisance in my life that I would consider not having children because of my fear of passing on this torment to a child.

What is the risk of my child having migraine?

ANSWER: Unfortunately, there is no uniform genetic marker or specific body fluid test to identify all migraineurs. The inheritance pattern of migraine is far from clear. It is known that individuals with identical genetic makeup (identical or monozygotic twins) are more likely to both suffer from migraines than is the case with genetically dissimilar twins (nonidentical or dizygotic). Therefore, a complex mode of inheritance must be considered. However, some studies have suggested that the risk of a child of a migraineur being afflicted with migraine is 45%; this number would increase to 70% if both parents have migraine.

QUESTION: *I have been told that I have classic migraine. My aura consists of wavy lines and other peculiar visual changes. If I take subcutaneous Sumatriptan early in the aura, will this affect the course of the aura and/or headache?*

ANSWER: This issue was recently addressed in an article in *Neurology* and consisted of a controlled study performed by doctors in England, Germany, Norway, and Denmark. This study did not find any significant alteration in nature or duration of the migraine or subsequent headache if 6 mg of Sumatriptan was injected subcutaneously during an aura (*Neurology,* 44: 1487–1592, 1994).

QUESTION: *My doctor tells me that because my headaches are invariably on the same side, it's very possible that I have a brain tumor or another serious abnormality on the side of my headaches. He tells me that migraine never affects just one side. What should I do?*

ANSWER: Past generations of neurologists have used the invariable laterality sign as an indication of a structural process, that is, tumor or abnormal blood vessel, causing the patient's headaches. Studies have indicated approximately 20% of patients with super migraines have their headaches always on the same side. If you have never had an MRI scan, I would recommend this at some point.

QUESTION: *I have suffered migraines for most of my adult life. During my recent pregnancy, my migraines almost completely stopped. After delivery, however, my headaches are back with a vengeance. Imitrex has been helpful in the past for me; however, I am breast-feeding now. Is it safe to take Imitrex?*

ANSWER: It is known that Imitrex has been identified in the breast milk of animals. We have no information, unfortunately, about this in humans. Until there is evidence of Imitrex's safety in nursing women, this medication should probably be avoided.

QUESTION: *I'm a 34-year-old woman who suffers from migraine attacks, as well as from bulimia. Is there a connection?*

ANSWER: A recent publication has suggested there may be a link between the two illnesses. Of the thirty-four migraine patients surveyed in an eating disorder clinic, 88% admitted dieting, 59% admitted to food binging, and 26% reported having induced vomiting at some point in their life.

The migraineurs also scored high on half of the Eating Disorder Inventory Questionnaire, particularly with regard to body dissatisfaction, perfectionism, interpersonal distrust, and ineffectiveness. The authors conclude that a possible biochemical disorder may be involved. (For more information on causes of migraines, read chapter 2.)

QUESTION: *I know my headaches are related to food allergies. Really, I'm allergic to everything. My doctor is treating me with medications and other stuff, which I know will never work. I'm having severe headaches and missing work several times a month. What should I do?*

ANSWER: As we've discussed elsewhere in this book, the issue of food allergy-related migraine is very complex and controversial. We do feel that food allergy can play a role in migraine, but on a fairly infrequent basis.

The best approach for a migraine syndrome is to keep an open mind and be thorough with regard to exploring all possible factors that might be contributing to the frequency and severity of your headaches. If you are convinced that a particular treatment is not going to help you, then you will probably be right because of your negative attitude. Having a positive attitude about a new treatment is very important.

QUESTION: *My cat has frequent spells in which she vomits, becomes listless or irritable, and hides under the bed. These spells can last from twelve to twenty-four hours. Could my cat have migraine?*

ANSWER: This is certainly an interesting question. We are not aware of migraines existing in any type of animal, although animals do share other illnesses with humans. As we have described previously, the diagnosis of migraine is based primarily on history, and of course that is not available in this case, since the cat can't provide a detailed (or any!) history.

It is true that many mammals often are afflicted with neurologic disease similar to those of humans, including stroke and seizures. However, we have performed a literature search of the National Library of Medicine and been unable to find any reference to migraine in animals.

QUESTION: *I have both migraine and epilepsy and am on several different medications to treat the two conditions. Is there any way that my medication regimen can be simplified so that I don't have to take five medications, including some that might be good for my migraine but could make my seizures worse?*

ANSWER: It is fairly well accepted that some association exists between migraine and epilepsy. This recognition has important implications for physicians treating patients with either diagnosis. On one hand, a patient with epilepsy should be questioned extensively about possibly concurrent headaches; on the other hand, the migraine patient should be questioned about possible symptoms of epilepsy.

A recent powerful study conducted by Ottman and Lipton has confirmed a close connection between epilepsy and migraines, but did not explain the nature of the association. There does not appear to be any relationship between the type of seizures, their cause, the patient's age at first seizure, or even family history of seizures and migraines.

As we mentioned previously, valproic acid (Depakote) appears to be helpful for both conditions. This medication is not good for all types of seizures but certainly is an effective tool in the management of many cases of epilepsy.

Moreover, it seems to decrease the frequency and severity of migraine attacks. Certainly a patient with migraines should avoid tricyclic medications as they could potentially make your seizures worse.

QUESTION: *I have heard about a new test for diagnosing migraine called transcranial doppler. Should I have this test done?*

ANSWER: Probably not. Transcranial doppler (TCD) is a method to study the arterial blood supply of the brain. By sending pulses of sound waves into the skull from various sites, the echo can be analyzed to provide some information about the speed of blood flow.

At least one study has suggested that the blood flow velocities in migraineurs is markedly increased. While this is certainly interesting, its diagnostic implications at this point are unresolved. Performing a TCD in a suspected migraine patient is, at this point, still experimental.

QUESTION: *Can the visual changes which occur in patients with migraine headache disorder be permanent?*

ANSWER: While permanent visual changes are very infrequent, it is true that persistent visual phenomena occur in rare individuals who suffer from migraine headache disorder. This problem can last from weeks to months and even up to years. As was recently reported in the April 1995 *Neurology Journal* (the premiere journal for neurology specialists), these phenomena occur in select and unfortunate individuals.

Oftentimes, people will seek the attention of an ophthalmologist (eye doctor) prior to realizing that these are indeed related to their migraine headache syndrome. If the visual disturbance persists, medical attention should be sought.

QUESTION: *When should I be concerned about my headache?*

ANSWER: Headaches are a sign of an underlying illness process and should always merit your attention. However, as neurologists, we feel that headaches are of concern primarily if they meet certain criteria, which include the following:

- The worst headache ever
- A sudden thunderclap or immediate onset of headache, which becomes intractable
- Headache symptoms that first occur after the age of 45
- Headaches associated with progressive severity
- Headaches associated with neurologic signs or symptoms, which would include numbness, weakness, tingling, burning, stumbling, falling, loss of balance or coordination, and severe visual changes
- Headaches that worsen with cough, sneeze, or straining with a bowel movement
- Any headache that concerns you, particularly if it follows an atypical course or persists for more than 24–36 hours

QUESTION: *My doctor, who has worked with me for some time, has suggested a headache center for my problem with frequent headaches. Do these clinics help?*

ANSWER: Patients are often referred to us for an inpatient evaluation. That means, we decide whether or not to admit patients to the hospital for management of their severe headache disorder. While a comprehensive team approach with the specialist, psychologist, social worker, exercise physiologist, and physical therapist is often helpful, we use inpatient therapy and hospital admission only as a last resort.

Frequently, a careful medical history will provide valuable clues for treating and resolving your severe headache syndrome. Also, it is important that you keep an accurate headache diary, an example of which can be found in the Appendix.

QUESTION: *How long after I change my diet and follow a specific headache diet should I see results?*

ANSWER: This is difficult to determine. As noted elsewhere in this book, some migraine sufferers will only have a headache every three to six months, and others will have a headache even less frequently.

We feel that a headache elimination diet of triggers will take anywhere from 6 to 12 weeks before one could even begin to assess its true efficacy. However, in certain individuals, a headache diet takes even longer to be completely effective, and it is more a matter of degree than an all-or-none phenomenon.

If you are getting some benefit with your diet, and there is any reduction in severity, intensity, or frequency of your headaches, we urge that you "stick with it."

QUESTION: *I have been reading in some magazines that one of the treatments for migraine is to replace magnesium. Can I* *give myself a magnesium injection, and how do I go about doing this?*

ANSWER: While you are correct in your assumption that magnesium may place a role in the production and ultimately termination of migraine headache pain, we strongly urge our patients to avoid self-medication until we know exactly whether or not their magnesium level is low.

We don't allow our patients to provide magnesium injections. Instead, these injections must be provided by a physician. Often, when a low magnesium level has been detected, we will allow our patients to take a multivitamin supplement with magnesium as part of the supplement.

If there is any question as to whether or not you have a low magnesium level, your physician certainly can draw a blood test to assess this.

QUESTION: *I have heard that there are medicines that can be taken as a nasal spray to terminate migraine headaches. Can you tell me what these are, and how do they act?*

ANSWER: There are a few intranasal medication treatments, the most common being Stadol nasal spray (butorphanol). This acts as a narcotic medication to manage the headache pain, which can often be successful in terminating a migraine headache.

In addition, this is often successful in combination with other medication, particularly as a secondary medication (such as after an Imitrex injection). Additional medications that are useful in the nasal form are dihydroergotamine nasal spray. (This medication is not yet available in the U.S. but is used widely with promising results in other countries.)

Other preparations may soon be available for specific termination of migraine headache pain. Please consult your physician as to the exact dosage for your height and weight and medical history.

QUESTION: *If I have a headache disorder, does that mean that I need to have a picture of my brain (CAT scan or other study)?*

ANSWER: No. Most people who have common migraine headache disorders rarely need to undergo special imaging studies (CAT scan, x-rays, magnetic scans of the brain or neck).

Unless your headache involves other signs or symptoms such as numbness, incoordination, clumsiness, tingling, burning, weakness, or dizziness, you most likely can be followed clinically. Nevertheless, this is something you should discuss with your physician, particularly after reviewing a complete medical history.

QUESTION: *Can poor sleeping habits play some role in my frequent recurrent headaches?*

ANSWER: Absolutely. One of the issues which we discuss in our chapter on lifestyle changes is controlling your sleep cycle, and we have provided multiple clues as to how to do this.

We feel that the expression "If only I could get a good night's sleep, I know I would feel better" is certainly not an old wives' tale. We feel that good sleep is absolutely mandatory to effect a positive change in patients who suffer from migraine headaches. We often prescribe sleep medications, such as Ambien, to help patients adjust their sleep cycle and hopefully return their sleep pattern to normal.

QUESTION: *My dentist told me I have TMJ. Can this be playing any role in my headaches?*

ANSWER: Definitely. In addition, many people do not know that they are grinding their teeth (bruxism) during sleep. Oftentimes, a simple bite block or mouthpiece, which can be fitted for individual patients and worn at nighttime, can prevent the jaw grinding, thereby reducing the jaw pain, the TMJ pain, and subsequently the risk of daily headaches.

The mechanism of action of jaw joint pain producing headaches is one that is related to the muscle contraction theory of headache. When the muscles over the jaw joints go into spasm, they trigger other muscles to tighten up, causing contraction of muscles along the base of the skull, the back of the neck, and into the shoulders.

This then produces triggers, waste toxins, and waste products, and leads to severe head and neck pain. This can be a vicious cycle and certainly needs to be addressed. A competent dentist and maxillofacial surgeon (dental specialist in jaw alignment) can often alleviate this problem without the use of medications, and can often break the headache cycle promptly.

QUESTION: *My husband smokes, and I tell him to stop it. I always seem to do worse when he smokes and I wonder if his smoking can be playing any role in my headaches.*

ANSWER: Yes. Women are more susceptible to cigarette smoke as a trigger than men, and in addition, are more susceptible to chemicals, odors, and perfumes that may act as triggers for their severe headache and migraine pain.

Additional triggers and precipitating factors for migraine that are more common in women than in men include the following: weather changes, missed meals, perfume, cigarette smoke, sunlight, stress, and sleeping too little. Triggers that are more common in men than in women include headaches associated with exercise and with sexual activity.

QUESTION: *How can I identify what is causing my headache?*

ANSWER: This is a complex question that is discussed in several chapters of this book. However, briefly, we offer the following advice:

- Keep a headache diary.

- Ask friends and family members to comment regarding moods, behaviors, and activities that occur immediately before or during headache attacks.

- Chart cycles in your headache, including their relationship to the weekdays vs. weekends, the menstrual cycle (if you are a woman), payday, and so on. Monitor your diet, activity, and sleep cycle. Then discuss all the above information with your physician, to see if together you can find your headache triggers and determine an effective treatment.

QUESTION: *I have my headaches at the time of my menstrual cycle. Is there anything in particular that is helpful for this?*

ANSWER: Yes. As we have discussed elsewhere in this book, many women will suffer what is called catamenial migraine. There is actually very specific treatment for certain individuals who have this, which includes the following:

Anti-inflammatory medications

Ergotamine preparations

Dihydroergotamine

Methergine

Methysergide

Standard preventative medicines such as tricyclic medications (Elavil, Pamelor), calcium channel blockers (verapamil, Calan, etc.), beta-blockers (Inderal, Tenormin, Lopressor).

Parlodel is often very effective for catamenial migraine, although this medicine is much more commonly used in patients with Parkinson's disease.

In addition, we have had very good success with Diamox, a type of water pill, which can reduce the swelling and the bloating of menses, as well as prevent a migraine headache.

If these medications are not effective, some authorities will recommend using stronger medicines such as steroid medications, as well as tranquilizers. We try to avoid these in our practice.

QUESTION: *Who treats migraine headaches?*

ANSWER: Oftentimes, general practitioners and family physicians will attempt to initiate the treatment and management of headache pain. However, if the pain syndrome requires medications, physician visits, and is involved with any type of lifestyle change or medical disability, the specialist who treats headache disorders (migraine and non-migraine headaches) is a neurologist.

Neurologists are specialists who deal with the central and peripheral nervous system, that is, the brain, the spinal cord, the nerve roots, the nerve twigs, and the muscles that are supplied by these.

The Academy of Neurology, an excellent resource, as well as other agencies helpful in answering questions regarding headache disorders, are listed in the Appendix.

QUESTION: *I tend to have more migraines when I travel. Why is this?*

ANSWER: There are many reasons for this. When we travel, we all tend to change our routine activities and get out of our normal lifestyle pattern. We seem to have changes in our appetite, our eating behaviors, and the foods we eat.

In addition, our sleep cycle is often changed or deranged entirely. Our exercise activity is quite different than in our home and natural environment. Often when we travel, we are exposed to changes in altitude and climates, as well as temperature changes.

Another point to keep in mind is that to arrive at a destination, we often travel by car, train, or airplane, and are exposed to various motions, all of which can act as migraine triggers. It is rarely one isolated aspect of the travel that produces these triggers, so identifying carefully all aspects that seem to play a role can often lead to alleviating this phenomenon.

QUESTION: *Can yeast infections cause migraines?*

ANSWER: Any stress to the body can act as a trigger for migraine pain. Patients who have upper respiratory infections or influenza, women who are menstruating, and individuals under psycho-social stressors are all more susceptible to migraine syndrome.

One popularly held theory is that this yeast infection is actually a connection to the immune system, acting to trigger our immune response and start this cascade effect, which we discuss under "Theories of Migraine." Another concept is that the yeast connection acts as a variant of an allergic reaction where the body initiates an allergic response at some level to trigger headache disorders. While yeast infections may indeed be a trigger in certain individuals, the jury is still out as to what the complete role of yeast infections in migraine pain disorders truly is.

QUESTION: *My doctor has recommended that I get a shot to treat my headache pain. Do you know what he is talking about, and how would this work?*

ANSWER: We are not exactly sure which type of shot your physician is recommending. As a general overview, perhaps the following will be helpful:

We use different types of injections for managing not only migraines but also daily headache pain syndromes. Of course, this is not our first choice of therapy.

Some injections are simply narcotic injections for the pain management. Narcotics comes from the Greek word "narcos," which means "to sleep," and the narcotic injection will simply put the pain to sleep for a short period of time. We prefer not to use these, as these can be habit-forming and addicting. They are often effective, but frequently will have significant side effects.

Additional injections include medicines given through the vein, such as intravenous magnesium or intravenous medicines to prevent nausea and to produce sleep. These have been discussed elsewhere in this book.

Other injections provide a neuroblockade (blockage of the pain messengers and the pain information transmission from the brain throughout the rest of the body). These often include medications that produce anesthesia (such as xylocaine or lidocaine, which most patients receive as they get a dental procedure), and are fairly well tolerated.

Neuroblockade injections frequently produce only a period of anesthesia or numbness. The numbing medication may often be given with a second injection, that being a steroid-type medication, which can provide a long-acting anti-inflammatory effect, preventing inflammation in the muscles, ligaments, tendons, and joints that often are secondary phenomena from muscle spasm and muscle contractions.

These injections are often given at the base of the skull, as well as in the mid-portion of the back of the neck. The Academy of Anesthesiology often recommends that these be administered as a series of three shots, but we suggest that our patients have a trial of an initial injection, and if this works, then a second and third injection may be helpful.

Finally, local trigger injections, often with just local anesthetic agents such as xylocaine or lidocaine or marcaine, are helpful to alleviate pain at an isolated trigger point. All of these therapies are best discussed with your physician and indeed even better discussed with a specialist who performs these pain injections, such as an individual who has completed a fellowship in pain management.

QUESTION: *I have frequent sick headaches. My doctor does not seem to take them seriously and often states: "Well, here's a different medication." What can I do to convince my doctor that these are disabling, and how do I go about getting rid of my headaches?*

ANSWER: This is a complex question, as we have discussed elsewhere in this book. However, briefly, in the doctor/patient relationship, you bring the most important aspect—the patient. It is important that you provide accurate and concise information regarding your symptom complex.

Nevertheless, if you cannot convince your physician to appreciate the severity of your illness, or if you do not feel that you and your physician are communicating effectively, as we have stated early in chapter 8 on "Choosing the Right Doctor," it is probably time to find a new or additional physician, one who has particular interest or expertise in treating patients who suffer from headache disorders.

Also, it would be helpful to present your new doctor with a comprehensive headache diary, one that demonstrates how different aspects of your life and lifestyle are affected by your headaches. This would include information regarding diet, exercise, activity, sleep cycle, work cycle, days missed from work, and activities that had to be changed or canceled because of your headache pain. This often is effective in convincing your physician that this is indeed "a serious problem."

QUESTION: *I have suffered from migraines, and now my 9-year-old son has apparently developed a migraine headache disorder. Are there different medicines for him than there are for me?*

ANSWER: Actually, the medication management for migraine in young children is somewhat different than it is for adults. While many physicians like to use Inderal, a relatively safe and effective medication for the prevention of migraine, it does indeed have some side effects. Also, this is a medication that should be avoided in children with asthma.

Nevertheless, oftentimes behavior modification, removal of triggers, and change in lifestyle patterns can be effective in alleviating the migraine disorder in children, and this can alleviate the need for medication management. In addition, it is important to recognize that migraines in children may be experienced as abdominal discomfort, malaise, fatigue, and a general sense of being unwell, and may not present with the complete spectrum of a migraine disorder that adults seem to experience.

This should be discussed with your pediatrician, and possibly a neurologist or pediatric neurologist would be helpful in evaluating your son's condition.

QUESTION: *My eye doctor told me that my vision changes could be a migraine attack. How could this be and what do I do for it?*

ANSWER: Your eye doctor may be right. Ophthalmic migraines are not uncommon, although permanent effects from ophthalmic migraines are quite rare. The diagnosis for ophthalmic/retinal migraine includes reversible single eye blindness or vision changes lasting less than 60 minutes, with the patient able to clearly identify a visual disturbance and draw the visual disturbance.

The headache will often follow the visual symptoms within 60 minutes, but may indeed precede the visual disturbance. There is an entirely normal eye examination away from the attack. This may be due to spasm or reduction in the blood flow to the retinal artery (the artery that supplies blood and oxygen to the eye), and there may be swelling of the artery wall. Standard anti-migraine therapy such as beta-blockers, calcium channel blockers, and aspirin therapy are often quite helpful. This condition should be discussed with your physician.

Appendix 1:
Activities for Daily Living

❖❖❖ ❖❖❖ ❖❖❖

This section includes basic and helpful advice for migraineurs, as well as people who suffer from muscle contraction headaches.

The following section will discuss proper body mechanics for your daily activities. In some cases, the mechanical stresses (load) to the spine for various positions has been included. This will give you an understanding of the importance of adequate strength, flexibility, and proper alignment in order to: (1) reduce load, (2) improve function, (3) alleviate pain and discomfort, and (4) prevent further injury.

The standard mechanical stress load to the spine is 100 percent when standing with correct posture.

Walking Posture

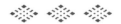

As you begin to walk, consciously pull your head, neck, and shoulders back. Heel should strike first while pushing off with the toes of the back foot. As you step forward, lift trunk tall and pull abdominals in.

This may feel strange at first, but remember you are not used to walking or moving with correct alignment. Eventually this will feel natural.

Prolonged Standing Technique

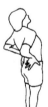

While standing for prolonged periods of time, stagger feet shoulder width apart and shift weight from one leg to the other. To alleviate pressure on the lower back while ironing or doing dishes, stand close to the ironing board or sink with one leg elevated 2 to 4 inches off the floor. Avoid leaning forward from the pelvis, back, or shoulders.

NOTE: Keep a soft knee, abdominals in, shoulders back, and raised sternum (breast bone). Keep your head and neck back.

Frequent One-Minute Breaks

The one-minute break is designed to enable you to change position frequently. Take time to get up and move around. Perform a few of the exercises you have learned. Use the corner stretch to help you stretch the chest and straighten your posture. Walk around your desk or office. Go to the bathroom.

Do anything that gets you moving.

Using the Telephone

When talking on the telephone, keep your head level, with shoulders and neck back.

Try not to hold the telephone with your shoulder elevated and head tilted to the side. This holds stress and tension in the upper back and neck.

Sleeping

Improper sleeping posture increases the mechanical stress on the spine. The tightness in the soft tissues of the pelvis and legs, coupled with poor hip alignment, can be a source of discomfort along the whole spine. This can lead to neck spasm. The following rules will aid in supporting the spine and pelvis as well as reducing the mechanical stress to the spine.

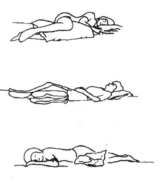

1. Sleep on a firm mattress to reduce tension caused by excessive curvature.
   - If you sleep on your side: place a pillow in between your knees. This will reduce the mechanical stress to 75%.
   - If you sleep on your back: place a pillow under your knees. This will reduce the mechanical stress to 5%. With legs extended, stress increases to 150%.
   - If you sleep on your abdomen: place a pillow underneath your hips.

Ideal Sitting and Driving Posture

Sitting causes the greatest increase in spine pressure (up to 275 percent); therefore, proper sitting posture is essential in order to reduce chronic back pain. Knees should be slightly higher than the hips, and your back should be firmly supported by the back of the chair or seat. The chair back should ideally be on an incline and have arm rests.

Keep head and neck retracted and abdominals in. While driving, keep both hands on the steering wheel, in the 10 and 2 o'clock positions, for support. Be certain that you are close enough to the foot pedals so that you do not have to reach for them.

Note: Sit in correct posture. Adjust all mirrors to accommodate this posture. The mirrors will act as a reminder to correct your position when your posture fails. Also, place a rolled towel in the natural curve of your lower back to add support and to remind you to remain in correct posture.

Mechanical Stress to the Low Back:
Sitting with Proper Posture: 140 percent
Sitting with Improper Posture: up to 275 percent

GETTING OUT OF BED OR OFF THE COUCH

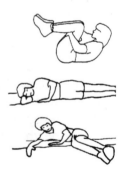

Using proper mechanics to get out of bed will reduce unnecessary tension on the spine. Before getting out of bed, bring knees to chest and grasp legs under knees. Pull into chest and raise shoulders to meet knees. Hold 10 to 30 seconds, release, then repeat. This will help you get ready to move. Roll onto your side and use your free arm to help push your torso up while you simultaneously swing your feet and legs off the bed or couch. This will leave you in a seated position.

STANDING AND SITTING

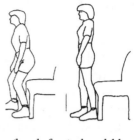

Using the proper technique to stand and/or sit will strengthen the legs and reduce discomfort and stress on the vertebrae.

To stand: Move to the edge of the chair. Place feet shoulder-width apart with one foot slightly in front of the other (back foot should be placed slightly under chair). Lean forward from the hips. Lift body with your legs. Stand erect and in good posture.

To sit: Stand tall with shoulder blades squeezing together. Back calf against the chair. Feet should be shoulder-width apart with one foot slightly in front of the other foot. Pull abdominals in, push hips back, and bend knees. Using the legs, ease back into the chair.

GETTING IN AND OUT OF A CAR OR CONFINED SPACE

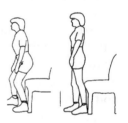

Always get in and out of a car without twisting or separating the legs. This leaves the pelvis in an unsupported position—increasing the mechanical stress on the spine. To get into a car, turn your body so that your back is facing the seat. Use proper sitting technique to sit in the car seat, then swing both legs into the car simultane-

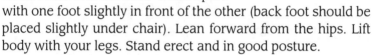

ously. Getting out of the car is the exact opposite. Begin by moving both legs out of the car (using a full body turn). Place one foot in front of the other, lean forward from the hips, and stand erect. Keep shoulders back and chest elevated.

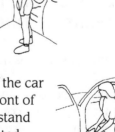

Half Kneeling

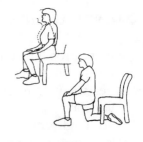

Move to the edge of your chair. Place one foot in front of the other with back leg under chair. With back flat and abs in tight, lean forward from the hips while pressing through the heel on your front leg, lift up and back onto the chair. This technique is great for getting clothes out of the dryer, getting things out of low cabinets, and so on.

Getting Off the Floor

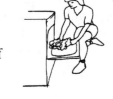

Half kneeling is a precursor to getting off the floor.

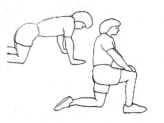

Roll onto all fours. Pull abdominal muscles in tight, walk hands back toward knees, and move into a kneeling position using your bent leg for support. You can now get into a chair or stand straight up using the half-kneeling technique.

Proper Lifting and Transporting Techniques

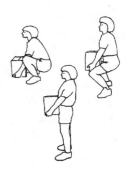

Lifting in any position will increase the mechanical load on the spine. The mechanical advantage to lifting with proper technique is to reduce the compressive forces on the spine and increase the stability of the spine during lifting and transport.

8. Have you had any diagnostic testing thus far?
   a. X-rays
   b. CT brain
   c. MRI brain
   d. EEG
   e. Laboratory tests
   f. Other:

9. Have you gone more than 3 months at a time without any headaches?

10. Have you tried any nonmedical treatments for your migraine:
    a. Herbal/nontraditional medicines
    b. Stress management techniques
    c. Exercise
    d. Yoga/meditation
    e. Breathing techniques
    f. Other:

11. Is there any relationship between work activities and your headaches (such as sitting at a chair, doing manual labor, etc.)?

12. If the answer to #11 was yes, what is the relationship?

13. Do you have a good sleep cycle?

14. If the answer to #12 is no, do you have trouble:
    a. Falling asleep
    b. Maintaining sleep
    c. Awakening too early

15. Have you ever had a problem with habit-forming medications?

16. How long was the longest headache you've experienced?

17. How short was the shortest headache you've experienced?

18. Do you have any unusual components to your headache:
    a. Vision changes
    b. Nausea
    c. Disorientation
    d. Weakness/numbness
    e. Other:

19. Are you concerned that your headaches represent a "brain tumor"?

GLOSSARY

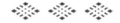

abnormal blood vessels. An abnormal connection between arteries and veins or an abnormal artery with an outpouching, leading to a weakened vessel and possible hemorrhage.

acupuncture. An Eastern style of therapy which uses special treatments of pressure and trigger points to release the body's own pain chemicals.

adrenaline. The body's stress chemical, which plays a role in our "fight or flight" natural instinct.

angiography. The study of a blood vessel from inside the artery; often a cousin to cardiac catheterizations, which look at the heart. Carotid and cerebral angiography look at the arteries of the neck and arteries of the brain, respectively.

antidepressants. Medications to reduce or relieve depression.

anti-emetics. Medicines that work to prevent or reduce nausea and vomiting.

aura. The premonition and sensation that a migraine headache will be following.

beta-blockers. A class of medicine that is used in migraine headache management. This is also used for blood pressure control and other illnesses.

breathing techniques. A special type of breathing pattern used to modulate pain and modulate and adjust the nervous system.

calcium channel blockers. A class of medicine used in migraine headache management, high blood pressure, and heart disease.

CAT scan. Computerized axial tomography scan, often used as a screening study to rule out hemorrhage in the brain and rule out brain tumor.

catamenial migraine. A unique type of migraine suffered by women that occurs at the time of menstruation.

chronic daily headaches. Headaches that occur on a daily basis, usually not migraine headaches.

classic migraine. A migraine headache associated with a warning or premonition, often a vision disturbance.

cluster headaches. A certain type of headache disorder.

common migraine. Migraine headache not associated with a warning or premonition and not associated with any visual disturbance.

diathermy. The use of ice and heat in pain management.

diuretic. Water pill.

emergency headache. A headache that demands emergency attention.

endorphins. The body's natural pain chemicals, produced in the brain.

guided imagery. Similar to hypnosis and breathing techniques; used as a method to adjust the nervous system and produce relaxation.

hypnosis. A unique type of focused attention, often effective in adjusting the body's heart rate, pulse, breathing pattern, and pain levels.

homeopathic medications. Natural chemicals, often available in health food stores and frequently prescribed by holistic or homeopathic physicians; considered natural treatments for various ills.

hypoglycemia. Low blood sugar.

lumbar puncture. Spinal tap; a study used to check the spinal fluid contents to rule out hemorrhage, infection, or cancer.

meningitis. Inflammation and possible infection of the coverings of the brain and spinal cord (as in "spinal meningitis").

migraineur. A patient who suffers from migraine headaches.

monoamine oxidase inhibitors. A class of medicine used to alleviate depression. This class is also often effective in preventing migraine headaches.

MRI. Magnetic resonance imaging scan; a more elaborate image of the brain, which identifies the brain stem, the balance center of the brain, and the small folds of the brain. Scarring and small strokes are often better seen on MRI studies than on CAT scans.

MSG. Monosodium glutamate; one type of food additive that often is a trigger found in multiple foods (please see comments on food restriction and headache disorder).

neural. Pertaining to the nerves and nervous system.

neuro-blockade. Some form of chemical intervention to block the chemical transmitters of the brain and prevent headache.

neurochemical transmission depletion theory. A theory currently held, which is used to explain migraine and its complete spectrum of symptoms.

neurovascular. Pertaining to the nerves and blood vessels in combination.

nonpharmacologic treatments. Treatments for migraine headaches that do not utilize prescription medications.

NSAIDS. Nonsteroidal/anti-inflammatory drugs. Motrin is in this class of drugs, as are many other newer medications.

occipital neuralgia. Inflammation of the nerve at the base of the skull that goes up the back of the head and around the ear. This can lead to sharp, shooting, lacerating pains that can be mistaken for migraine or muscle spasm headaches.

prodrome. The events that precede a migraine headache; often these include nausea, queasiness, vision changes, and throbbing temples.

progressive relaxation. A method of contracting and relaxing a series of muscles in a progressive fashion, producing an overall sense of relaxation and calm.

pseudotumor cerebri. Increased pressure on the brain, often seen in overweight females and often associated with vision problems.

serotonin. A brain chemical that is often implicated in migraine headache disorder.

sinusitis. Inflammation and possible infection of the sinus cavities.

stroke. Loss of blood and oxygen in the brain tissue, which leads to a loss of function related to that area of brain damage (such as weakness, numbness, clumsiness, loss of speech, or paralysis).

subcutaneous. Beneath the skin.

temporal arteritis. Inflammation of the arteries at the sides of the head. If left untreated, can lead to blindness.

tension headaches. The older term for muscle spasm/muscle contraction type headaches. These may be worse when the patient is under stress.

therapeutic massage. A unique type of massage that improves muscle spasm and contraction, as well as muscle inflammation, and is often effective for reducing muscle contraction and mixed headache disorders.

thermography. A temperature study of the brain.

TMJ. Temporomandibular joint dysfunction; these jaw joint problems may be related to headache pains.

transcranial doppler. A non-invasive ultrasound study of the brain's blood vessels.

trigeminal neuralgia. Often referred to as tic douloureaux; this is a brain stem nerve which causes pain in the face and can be confused with migraine or other types of headache pain.

trigger. An item or event that leads to a migraine headache.

tumor. An abnormal growth somewhere in the body, potentially a cancer growth.

tyramine. Chemical substance that acts as a potential chemical transmitter of the brain; may play a role in migraine headaches.

vascular. Pertaining to blood vessels.

visual aura. The flashes of light that precede a migraine headache.

BIBLIOGRAPHY

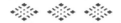

Alvarez, W. C. "The migrainous scotoma as studies in 618 persons." *American Journal of Ophthalmology,* 49:489–504, 1960.

American Academy of Allergy and Immunology. "Candidiasis hypersensitivity syndrome." *Journal of Allergy and Clinical Immunology,* 78:271–273, 1986.

Anthony, M. "Headache and the greater occipital nerve." *Clinical Neurology and Neurosurgery,* 94:297–301, 1992.

Appenzeller, O. "Pathogenesis of migraine (review)." *Medical Clinics of North America,* 75(3):763–789, May 1991.

Axon, M., et al. "Migraine angitis precipitated by sex headache and leading to watershed infarction." *Cephalgia,* 13:427–430, 1993.

Balch, J. F., et al. *Prescription for Nutritional Healing.* Garden City Park, New York: Avery Publishing Group, 1990.

Barlow, C. F. *Headaches and Migraines in Children.* Oxford: Spastics International Medical Publications, 1984.

Barnard, N. *Power of Your Plate.* Summer-Town, Tennessee: Book Publishing Company, 1990.

Baumel, B., et al. "Diagnosis and treatment of headache in the elderly." *Medical Clinics of North America,* 75:661–675, 1991.

Belgrade, M. J., et al. "Comparison of single dose Meperidine, Butorphanol, and Dihydroergotamine in the treatment of vascular headache." *Neurology,* 39:590–592, 1989.

Blanchard, E. B. "Behavioral therapies in the treatment of headache." *Headache Quarterly: Current Treatment and Research,* 1:53–56, 1993.

Blau, J. N. "How to take a history of head or facial pain." *British Medical Journal,* 285:9–1251, October 30, 1982.

Blau, J. N., et al. "The site of pain origin during migraine attacks." *Cephalgia,* 1:143–147.

Boggs, J. G., et al. "Migraine in liver transplant patients." *Neurology,* 45(supplement 4):A366, April 1995.

Bradley, Walter G., et al. *Neurology and Clinical Practice.* Boston: Butterworth-Heinemann, 1991.

Buring, J. E., et al. "Migraine and subsequent risk of stroke in the physician's health study." *Neurology,* 52:129–134, 1995.

Cantor, T. G. "Pharmacology and Mechanisms of Some Pain Relieving Drugs," *Headache Quarterly.* February 1988, 61–62.

Cantrell-Simmons, E., et al. "A review of studies on the relationship of chronic analgesic use in chronic headaches." *Headache Quarterly,* 4:28–35, 1993.

Carlsson, J., et al. "Muscle tenderness in tension headache treated with acupuncture or physiotherapy." *Cephalgia,* 10:131–141, 1990.

Castleman, M. *The healing herbs.* Emmaus, PA: Rodale Press, 1991.

Coyle, P. K. "Neurologic complications of Lyme disease and neurologic aspects of rheumatic disease." *Rheumatic Disease Clinics of North America,* 19(4):993–1009, November 1993.

Cronen, M. C., et al. "Cervical steroid epidural nerve block in the palliation of pain secondary to intractable muscle contraction headache." *Headache,* 28:314–315, 1988.

Cummings, Stephen, M.D., and Ullman, Dana, M.P.H. *Everybody's Guide to Homeopathic Medicines.* New York: Jeremy P. Tarcher/Putnam Book, 1991.

Dahlof, M. D., Ph.D., Ekbaum, K., M.D., Ph.D., and Persson, Lennart, M.D., Ph.D. "Clinical Experiences from Sweden on the Use of Subcutaneously Administered Sumatriptan in Migraine and Cluster Headache." *Archives of Neurology,* 51:1256–1261, December 1994.

Dalessio, D. J., et al. *Wolf's headache and other head pain.* Sixth Ed., New York: The University Press, 1993.

Dalessio, D. J. "On the safety of caffeine as an analgesic adjuvant." *Headache Quarterly: Current Treatment and Research,* 5(2):125–127, 1994.

Davidoff, R. A. *Migraine: Manifestations, pathogenesis and management.* Davis Company of Philadelphia, 1995.

DeMatteis, G., et al. "Geomagnetic activity, humidity, temperature and headache: Is there any correlation?" *Headache,* 34:41–43, 1994.

Diamond, S. "Diagnosis and treatment of migraine." *Clinical Journal of Pain,* 5:3–9, 1989.

Diamond S., et al. "Transnasal Butorphanol in the treatment of Migraine Head Pain." *Headache Quarterly,* 3:160–167, 1992.

Drugs for Migraine. *The Medical Letter,* 37(issue 943):17–20, March 3, 1995.

Ducro, P. N., et al. "Migraine as a sequel to chronic low back pain." *Headache,* 34:279–281, 1994.

Eger, J., et al. "Effective diet treatment on anuresis in children with migraine or hyperkinetic behavior." *Clinical Pediatrics,* (Philadelphia) 5:302–307, May 31, 1992.

Ermenda, P. D., et al. "Extracranial vascular changes as a source of pain in migraine headache." *Annals of Neurology,* 13:32–37, 1983.

Ferrari, M. D., et al. "Treatment of migraine attacks with Sumatriptan." *New England Journal of Medicine,* 325:316–321, 1991.

Ferrari, M. D., et al. "Cerebral blood flow during migraine attacks without aura and effect of Sumatriptan." *Neurology,* 52:135–139, 1995.

Freschi, Joseph R., "Why Migraine Headaches," *Total Health,* 15(6): 36 (2), December 1993.

Friberg, L., et al. "Cerebral oxygen extraction, oxygen consumption, and regional cerebral blood flow during the aura phase of migraine." *Stroke,* 25:974–979. 1994.

Gauthier, J., et al. "The role of home practice in the thermal biofeedback treatment of migraine headache." *Consult Clinical Psychology,* 62 (1):180–184, February 1994.

George, M. S. "Is migraine related to eating disorders?" *International Journal of Eating Disorders,* 14(1):75–79, July 1993.

Good, P. A., et al. "The use of tinted glasses in childhood migraine." *Headache,* 31:533–536, 1991.

Goulart, F. S. "The headache alternative: Fifteen natural pain-pain-go-away solutions." *Total Health,* 16, N3: 26(3), June 1994.

Grazzi, L., et al. "Italian experience of electromyographic biofeedback treatment of episodic common migraine: Preliminary results." *Headache,* 33:439–441, 1993.

Hainline, Brian. "Headache." *Neurologic Clinics,* 12(3), August 1994 (neurologic complications of pregnancy, 443–459).

Hay, K. M., et al. "1044 women with migraine: The effect of environmental stimuli." *Headache,* March 1994, 166–194.

HEADway, "Now there is MMS: Menstrual Migraine Syndrome." *Newsletter for migraine sufferers,* vol. 3.

Hofert, M. J. "Treatment of migraine: A new era (review)." *American Family Physician,* 49(3):633-638, 643–644, February 15, 1994.

Igarashi, M., et al. "Pharmacologic treatment of childhood migraine (review)." *Journal of Pediatrics,* 120(4, Part I):653–657, April 1992.

Inan, L. E., et al. "Complicated retinal migraine." *Headache,* 34:50–52, 1994.

Jensen, R. "Sodium valproate has a prophylactic effect in migraine without aura, a triple blind placebo-controlled crossover study." *Neurology,* 44:647–651, 1994.

Johnson, E. S., et al. "Efficacy of feverfew as prophylactic treatment of migraine." *British Medical Journal,* 291:569–573, 1985.

Jorgensen H. S., et al. "Headache And Stroke: The Copenhagen Stroke Study." *Neurology,* 44:1793–1797, 1994.

Kudro, L. "Paradoxical effects of frequent analgesic use." *Advances in Neurology,* 33, 1982, 335–341.

Lake, A. E., et al. "Comprehensive inpatient treatment for intractable migraine: A prospective long-term outcome study." *Headache,* 33(2):55–62, February 1993.

Lance, F. "Does analgesic abuse cause headaches de novo?" *Headache,* February 1988, 61–62.

Lauritzen, M. "Pathophysiology of the migraine aura. The spreading depression sere (review)." *Brain,* 117(Part I):199–210, February 1994.

Linet, M. S., et al. "An epidemiologic study of headache in adolescents and young adults." *JAMA,* 261:2211–2216, 1989.

Liu, G. T., et al. "Persistent positive visual phenomena in migraine." *Neurology,* 45:664–668, 1995.

Lundberg, P. O. "Abdominal migraine—Diagnosis and therapy." *Headache,* 15:122–125, 1975.

Mahaja, A. N., et al. "Platelet phospholipase inhibitor from the medicinal herb feverfew (tannacetum parthenium), prostaglandins, leukotrienes," *Medicine,* 8:653–660, 1982.

Mansfield, L. "Food allergy and migraine: Double blind and mediator confirmation of an allergic etiology." *Annals of Allergy,* 55:92; 126–129, 1985.

Matthew, N. "Valproate in the treatment of persistent chronic daily headache." *Headache,* 30:301,1990.

Mauskop, A. "Chronic daily headache—One disease or two? Diagnostic role of serum ionized magnesium." *Cephalgia,* 14(1):24–28, February 1994.

Mauskop, Alexander, et al. "Intravenous (IV) magnesium sulfate (MgSO4) relieves acute migraine (M) in patients (P) with low serum ionized magnesium levels (IMG2+)." *Neurology,* 45(supplement 4): A379, April 1995.

McGrady, A., et al. "Effective biofeedback—assisted relaxation on migraine headache and changes of cerebral blood flow velocity in the middle cerebral artery." *Headache,* 34(7):424–428, July-August 1994.

Mortimer, M. J., et al. "The prevalence of headache and migraine in atopic children: An epidemiologic study in general practice." *Headache,* 33(8):427–431, September 1993.

Moskowitz, M. A. "Brain mechanisms in vascular headache." *Neurologic Clinics,* 8:801–815, 1990.

Nappi, Giuseppe. "Oral Sumatriptan compared with placebo in the acute treatment of migraine." *Journal of Neurology,* 241:138–144, 1994.

Neurologic Clinics: Headache, 1 (2) B. Saunders Co., Russel C. Packard, M.D., Guest Editor, May 1983.

Newman, L. C., Lipton, R. B. and Soloman, S. "Hemicrania Continua: Ten New Cases in Review of the Literature." *Neurology,* 44: 2111–2114, 1994.

Nicolodi, M., et al. "Visceral pain threshold is deeply lowered far from the head in migraine." *Headache,* 34:12-19, 1994.

Niedermeyer, E. "Migraine-Triggered Epilepsy." *Clinical Electroencephalography,* 24:37–43, 1993.

Oldman, B. "Chronic pain and the search for alternative treatments." *Medical Association Journal,* 145(5):508–513, 1991.

Olesen, J. "Understanding the biologic basis of migraine." *New England Journal of Medicine,* 331(25): 1713–1714.

Osipova, V. "Psycho-autonomic approaches to migraine." *Functional Neurology,* 7(4):263–273, July-August 1992.

Osterhaus, J. T., et al. "Health care resource and lost labor costs of migraine headache in the United States." *Pharmaco-economics,* 2:67–76, 1992.

Ottman, R. and Lipton, R. B. "Comorbidity of Migraine and Epilepsy." *Neurology,* 44:2105–2110, 1994.

Packard, R. C. "Emotional aspects of headache." *Neurologic Clinics: Symposium on Headache,* 1:445–456, 1983.

Panayiotopoulos, C. P. "Elementary visual hallucinations in migraine and epilepsy." *Journal of Neurology, Neurosurgery and Psychiatry,* 57:1371–1374, 1994.

Pareja, J. A., et al. "Sunct syndrome in the female." *Headache,* 34:217–220, 1994.

Passchier, J. "A critical note on psycho-physiological stress research into migraine patients (review article)." *Cephalgia,* 3:194–198, 1984.

Perlmutter, D. *Life Guide—Your guide to a longer and healthier life."* Vol. 1, 2nd ed. Naples, Florida: Life Guide Press, 1994.

Perneger, T. V., et al. "Risk of kidney failure associated with the use of acetaminophen, aspirin, and nonsteroidal/anti-inflammatory drugs." *New England Journal of Medicine,* 331:167–169, 1994.

Pradaliera, et al. "Treatment review: Nonsteroidal/anti-inflammatory drugs in treatment and long-term prevention of migraine attacks." *Headache,* 28:550–557, 1988.

Raskin, N. H. "Repetitive intravenous Dihydroergotamine for the treatment of intractable migraine." *Neurology,* 34:245, 1984.

Raskin, N. H. "Acute and prophylactic treatment of migraine: Practical approaches and pharmacological rationale (review)." *Neurology,* 43(6 supplement 3):S39–42, June 1993.

Raskin, N. H. "Headache (review)." *Western Journal of Medicine,* 161(3): 299–302, September 1994.

Reik, L. "Lyme disease—Current therapy." In R. Johnson, M.D. (ed.), *Neurologic Disease,* 3rd ed. textbook. Philadelphia: B. C. Decker, 1990.

Robbins, L. D. "Cryotherapy for headache." *Headache,* 29:598–600, 1989.

Robbins, L. "Precipitating factors in migraine: A retrospective review of 494 patients." *ACHE,* pp. 214–216, April 1994.

Sacks, Oliver. *Migraine: Evolution of a Common Disorder.* Berkeley: University of California Press, 1970.

Schesse, J. "Acupuncture vs. Metoprolol in migraine prophylaxis: A randomized trial of trigger point inactivation." *Journal of Internal Medicine,* 235:451-456, 1994.

Schulman, E. A., et al. "Symptomatic and prophylactic treatment of migraine and tension type headache (review)." *Neurology,* 42 (3 supplement 2):16–21, March 1992.

Shadick, N. A., et al. "The long-term clinical outcomes of Lyme disease." *Annals of Internal Medicine,* 121:560–567, 1994.

Smeets, M. C. "Intracellular and plasma magnesium in familial hemiplegic migraine and migraine with and without aura." *Cephalgia,* 14(1):29–32, February 1994.

Soloman, S., et al. "Breaking the cycle of pain." *Medical World News,* December 1993.

Stewart, W. F., et al. "Prevalence of migraine headache." *JAMA*, 267 (1): 64–69, January 1, 1992.

Stewart, W. F., Ph.D, M.P.H. "Impact of Migraine." *Neurology*, 44 (supplement 4):S5, 1994.

Stewart, W. F., Ph.D., M.P.H., "Migraine Prevalence: A Review of Population-Based Studies," *Neurology*, 44 (supplement 4): S17–23, 1994.

Subcutaneous Sumatriptan International Study Group, "Treatment of migraine attacks with Sumatriptan." *New England Journal of Medicine*, 325:316-327, 1991.

Silberstein, S. D. "Headaches in women: Treatment of the pregnant and lactating migraineur." *Headache*, 33:533–540, 1993.

Solomon, G. D. "Pharmacology and use of headache medications." *Cleveland Clinic Journal of Medicine*, 57:627–635, 1990.

Silvestrini, M., et al. "Migraine in patients with stroke and anti-phospholipid antibodies." *Headache*, 33:421–426, 1993.

Sjaastad, O. O., et al. "Cervicogenic headache; the differentiation from common migraine. An overview." *Functional Neurology*, 6(2):93–99, 1991.

Somerville, B. W. "A study of migraine in pregnancy." *Neurology*, 22:824–828, 1972.

Strom, B. L. "Adverse reactions to over-the-counter analgesics taken for therapeutic purposes." *JAMA*, 272(23):1866–1867, December 21, 1994.

Touchon, J., et al. "A comparison of SC Sumatriptan and intranasal Dihydroergotamine (DHE) in the treatment of migraine." *Neurology*, 45(supplement 4):A378, April 1995.

Trotsky, M. B. "Neurogenic vascular headaches, food, and chemical triggers." *Ears, Nose and Throat Journal*, 73(4):228–230, 235–236, April 1994.

Value of heat and ice therapy (educational bulletin). Gulf Coast Spine Institute, May 1995.

Vaughan, T. R. "The role of food in the pathogenesis of migraine headache." *Clinical Review of Allergy*, 12(2):167–180, Summer 1994.

Vijayan, N. "Head band for migraine headache relief." *Headache*, 33:40–42, 1993.

Vincent, C. A. "The treatment of tension headache by acupuncture: A controlled single case designed with time series analysis." *Journal of Psychosomatic Research,* 34(5):553–561, 1990.

Weiss, E., and English, O. S. *Psychosomatic Medicine,* 2nd Ed., Saunders, 1949.

Whitcomb, D. C., et al. "Association of acetaminophen hepatotoxicity with fasting and ethanol abuse." *JAMA,* 272:1845–1850, 1994.

Wilkinson, M. "Migraine treatment: The British perspective (Magnesium in migraine. Results in a multicenter pilot study), *Fortschr Medizin,* 112(24):328–330, August 30, 1994.

Wilson, J., et al. "Spreading cerebral oligemia in classical and normal cerebral blood flow in common migraine." *Headache,* 22:242–249.

Woods, R. P., et al. "Bilateral spreading cerebral hypoperfusion during spontaneous migraine headache." *New England Journal of Medicine,* 31(25):1689–1692, November 22, 1994.

Yuanm. "Clinical application of point-through-point acupuncture." *Journal of Traditional Chinese Medicine,* 12.

Ziegler, D. K. "Dihydroergotamine nasal spray for the acute treatment of migraine." *Neurology,* 44:447-453, 1994.

Ziegler, D. K. "Dihydroergotamine nasal spray." *Neurology,* 45.

INDEX

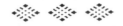

About the Authors

Joseph Kandel, M.D., is the founder and medical director of the Neurology Center of Naples, Florida, and cofounder of the Gulfcoast Spine Institute. An avid student since his youth, he attended Ohio State University as a Batelle Scholar, obtaining a double major B.S. in zoology and a B.S. in psychology, both with honors. Kandel graduated from Wright State University School of Medicine in Dayton, Ohio, in 1985, where he is now an associate clinical professor. He completed his neurology residency at the University of California Irvine Medical Center and is a Diplomate, American Board of Psychiatry and Neurology.

Kandel is a popular public speaker and has been published in such prestigious medical journals as *Neurology, Vital Signs,* and *American Zoologist.*

He lives in Naples with his wife and their three children.

David Sudderth, M.D., is the cofounder of the Gulfcoast Spine Institute and partner at Neuroscience and Spine Associates in Naples, Florida.

He graduated from medical school at the University of Copenhagen in 1984 and completed his residency at the Medical College of Wisconsin and Emory University. Dr. Sudderth accomplished a one-year fellowship in nerve and muscle disorders at Emory University in 1988.

An in-demand lecturer, Sudderth speaks frequently on medical topics. He also produced the popular video *Spinal Tips* and *Relief from Carpal Tunnel Syndrome.*

An avid computer fan, Dr. Sudderth can often be found perusing the Internet and other computer services, and will often answer questions from his webpage (www.neurologist.com).

Also by Drs. Kandel and Sudderth

Spinal Tips: Physician's Home Remedy for Back or Neck Pain
Videotape runs 46 minutes / $19.95 + $3.95 shipping and handling

> Chronic back and neck pain sufferers—you don't gain from pain!
> Get past the pain and enjoy your life again by following the ex-
> pert, practical, and immediately usable advice found in *Spinal
> Tips.* The video features simple exercises demonstrated by aver-
> age people (not athletes or sports specialists) that will help you
> feel markedly better!

***Relief from Hand and Arm Pain: Carpal Tunnel Syndrome
and Repetitive Stress Injuries***
Videotape runs 16 minutes / $14.95 + $3.95 shipping and handling

> Millions of people suffer from hand and wrist problems. If you are
> among them, this video can help greatly improve your problem or
> alleviate it all together! Drs. Kandel and Sudderth offer important
> preventive measures and easy exercises you can integrate into
> your daily life. Also included are valuable descriptions and
> demonstrations of tests doctors perform to detect repetitive stress
> injuries of the hand or wrist, as well as a discussion of surgical
> options.

Order from:

Pain Management Publishing
8380 Riverwalk Park Blvd., Suite 320
Fort Myers, FL 33907

For credit card orders, call 1-800-844-7880

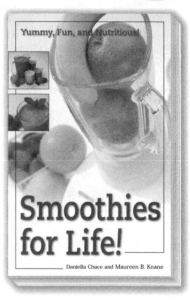

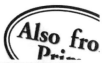
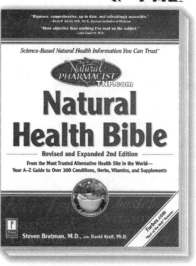

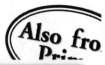

Interactions: The Dangers and Benefits

With the right vitamin or herb you can reduce or even eliminate certain side effects of many medications. On the other hand, taking the wrong vitamin or herb can increase some side effects or interfere with the effectiveness of medication.

   Inside, you'll learn how to reduce the risk of hazardous interactions and discover exactly which supplements to take to enhance the effectiveness of your medications. This book includes:

- **Detailed descriptions of drugs, herbs, and vitamins, and their uses**
- **A comprehensive guide to both negative and positive combinations**
- **Easy reference to specific drug-herb-supplement interactions**
- **And much more!**

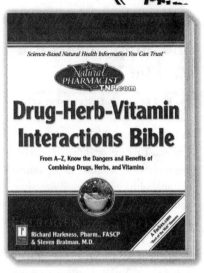

ISBN 0-7615-3013-4
Paperback / 448 pages
U.S. $19.99 / Can. $29.95

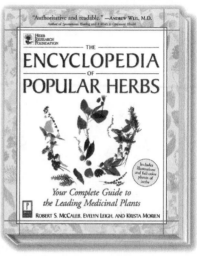